The Treatment of
Obesity

To my wife
who most appreciates how much weight I lost in editing this book

CURRENT STATUS OF MODERN THERAPY: VOLUME 2

The Treatment of
Obesity

Edited by
J. F. Munro

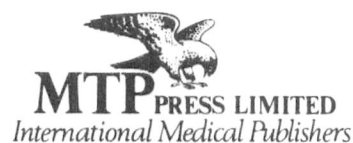

MTP PRESS LIMITED
International Medical Publishers

Published by
MTP Press Limited
Falcon House
Lancaster, England

Copyright © 1979 MTP Press Limited
Softcover reprint of the hardcover 1st edition 1979
First published 1979

British Library Cataloguing in Publication Data
The treatment of obesity. – (Current status of modern therapy; vol. 2).
  1. Obesity
  I. Munro, John Forbes   II. Series
  616.3'98'06   RC628
  ISBN 978-94-015-1134-6   ISBN 978-94-015-1132-2 (eBook)
  DOI 10.1007/978-94-015-1132-2

Contents

List of Contributors

R. M. BADDELEY
The General Hospital, Steelhouse Lane, Birmingham B4 6NH, England

P. BJÖRNTORP
Department of Medicine 1, Sahlgren's Hospital, University of Göteborg,
413 45 Göteborg, Sweden

J. E. BLUNDELL
Section of BioPsychology, Psychology Department, University of Leeds,
Leeds LS2 9JT, England

K. D. BROWNELL
Department of Psychiatry, University of Pennsylvania,
205 Piersol Building, Philadelphia, Pennsylvania 19104, USA

S. L. BURRIDGE
Section of BioPsychology, Psychology Department, University of Leeds,
Leeds LS2 9JT, England

M. J. FORD
The Royal Infirmary, Glasgow, Scotland

J. S. GARROW
Medical Research Council, Clinical Research Centre, Harrow HA1 3UJ,
England

A. N. HOWARD
Department of Medicine, University of Cambridge, Addenbrookes Hospital,
Hills Road, Cambridge, CB2 2QQ, England

A. C. MacCUISH
The Royal Infirmary, Glasgow, Scotland

J. F. MUNRO
   Edenhall Hospital, Musselburgh, Midlothian, Scotland

L. SJÖSTRÖM
   Department of Medicine 1, Sahlgren's Hospital, University of Göteborg,
   413 45 Göteborg, Sweden

A. J. STUNKARD
   Department of Psychiatry, University of Pennsylvania,
   205 Piersol Building, Philadelphia, Pennsylvania 19104, USA

L. SULLIVAN
   Department of Clinical Rehabilitation, Sahlgren's Hospital, University of
   Göteborg, 413 45 Göteborg, Sweden

Consultant Editor's Note

CURRENT STATUS OF MODERN THERAPY

The *Current Status of Modern Therapy* is a major series from MTP Press with the purpose of providing a definitive view of modern therapeutic practice in those areas of clinical medicine in which important changes are occurring. The series consists of monographs specially commissioned under the individual editorship of internationally recognized experts in their fields. Their selection of a panel of contributors from many countries ensures an international perspective on developments in therapy.

The series aims to review the growth areas of clinical pharmacology and therapeutics in a systematic way. It is a continuing series in which the same subject areas will be covered by revised editions as advances make this desirable.

Obesity is a fitting subject for the series for, although it is viewed in a different light within different cultures and in different ages, within our affluent society obesity is recognized as one cause of increased mortality. Hence for both cosmetic and medical reasons the treatment of obesity is accepted as important.

This latest volume in the Current Status of Modern Therapy Series – *The Treatment of Obesity* – shows that there is no single successful method of therapy for all patients, but it provides an excellent review of the latest ideas on this subject.

J. MARKS
Girton College
Cambridge

Series Editor

Preface

During the last few years, there has been growing medical interest in the problem of obesity. Although this may not have resulted in a dramatic breakthrough in our understanding of the condition, at least we are now more aware of our ignorance. Possibly this partly explains the increasing medical concern for, and sympathy in, the management of the obese. In the introductory chapter, John Garrow says that he believes it would be better to treat a few people well than many subjects unsuccessfully. This theme is developed in those chapters which deal with specific forms of therapy including exercise, protein-sparing fasting and bypass surgery, while the chapters on pharmacological agents review our knowledge, and our ignorance, of the mode of action and efficacy of the currently available drugs.

Almost in contrast, the chapter on behavioural therapy and group therapy suggests that obesity is a problem which could best be tackled on a community basis. Clearly such an approach is very attractive, and the combination of behavioural therapy and slimming organizations would appear to offer the best prospects of controlling most subjects' weight problems. There will always remain, however, the individual patient in whom there will be a place for the various special techniques now available.

It is hoped that this book will contribute to a greater understanding of the various problems faced by the obese, and the regimes that can be offered.

J. F. MUNRO

1

How to treat and when to treat

J. S. Garrow

INTRODUCTION

In theory it is obvious how to treat or prevent obesity: if it can be arranged that over the lifespan of an individual the total energy intake from food matches total energy expenditure, with suitable allowances for growth in childhood and for the physiological decrease in lean body mass in old age, then that individual cannot become obese. In practice this balance is often very difficult to achieve, and the medical literature is full of jeremiads about the impossibility of successful treatment. Astwood[1] said that obesity was due to an inborn error of metabolism, so people who are fat are born fat, and nothing much can be done about it. Kemp[2] said there is a point of no return at which the fat organ is so large that it becomes autonomous. Goldrick[3] questioned whether refractory obese patients should be treated at all.

Suggestions of this sort are dangerous nonsense. It is manifestly untrue that all fat people are born fat, since the majority of fat adults were not fat children[4]. Certainly some people have a greater predisposition to fatness than others, just as some people have a predisposition to diabetes or hypertension, but it is untrue that nothing much can be done about any of these diseases. Kemp's suggestion ignores the laws of thermodynamics, since however 'autonomous' the fat organ may be, it cannot increase its store of fat unless energy intake exceeds energy output. Most dangerous of all is the idea that 'refractory' obese patients should not be treated, since this is a classical example of the self-fulfilling prophecy: label a patient as refractory and withdraw treatment, and it is to be expected that his subsequent progress will justify the original diagnosis of 'refractory' obesity.

The disparity between the theoretical ease, and the actual difficulty, in treating obesity indicates a fundamental difference between this disease and others with which the average physician has to deal. It is the function

1

of doctors to make life more tolerable for their patients, and for many diseases the question 'How to treat and when to treat ?' does not arise. Any patient with a treatable disease is treated as and when the diagnosis is made. In general the reasons for *not* treating a patient are that by so doing the doctor would not achieve the objective of making life more tolerable for the patient. This situation arises either when the disease is too serious to cope with (as in terminal malignant disease), or too trivial (as in German measles), or when no useful treatment is known (as in multiple sclerosis). However, obesity does not fit into any of these categories: it is not a single disease. Indeed it is as unhelpful to talk about the treatment of 'obesity' as it would be about 'oedema', or 'jaundice'. The possible lines of treatment are discussed by other contributors to this volume: the purpose of this chapter is to discuss the factors which indicate which option is likely to provide the greatest benefit to a particular patient.

MOTIVATION AND EXPECTATION

The most important factor determining the success of treatment for obesity is the motivation and expectation of the doctor and patient. Probably most people who come to a doctor for treatment for obesity have already tried some line of treatment which has failed. The Consumers' Association received completed questionnaires from 2333 people who had tried by various means to lose weight[5]. Of these 1117 women and 245 men had received advice from a general practitioner, so roughly half of this sample had relied on slimming clubs, magazine articles and various commercial cures, and had not sought medical advice. It is difficult to assess the proportion of people who treat themselves and achieve satisfactory control of their weight, since obviously such statistics can only be obtained by interviewing random samples of the population. In the United States, polls of 5500 people in 1950, 1956 and 1966 showed that among men 21, 23 and 36% thought they were overweight, but in each year only 7% were actually dieting when interviewed[6]. The corresponding results for women were that 44, 45 and 42% thought they were overweight, and 14% said they were dieting when interviewed. In the light of these statistics it is naive to expect that an obese patient asking for medical advice will be greatly helped simply by a diet sheet. Any literate citizen of the United Kingdom can easily acquire advice on a reducing diet without bothering the doctor. If this was all that was required, the patient would not be seeing the doctor at all.

In the treatment of obesity, as with other complaints, it is necessary to find out what the patient is actually complaining about. The central problem usually presents in one of three forms, and it is necessary to establish to which category the patient belongs before any rational treatment is possible.

Probably the commonest problem encountered in a hospital obesity clinic is the patient who considers that her (for it is usually a woman) rate of weight loss is unreasonably slow. She observes other members of her family, or members of her slimming club, who lose weight far more rapidly than she does, and is sure that this is not because she eats more than her rivals. She may recall that in the past she easily lost 4 kg (9 lb) in a week, yet now she must fight hard to lose one or two pounds, and observes that on some days she actually gains weight. She may even report that her family doctor regards this as evidence of a disordered metabolism, which she wishes to have investigated. To cope with patients in this category it is necessary to have a clear understanding of the relationship between weight loss and energy deficit. It is convenient to think of the energy stores of the body in three compartments: adipose tissue, lean body mass, and a small and labile pool of glycogen and water. Adipose tissue is about 83% fat, 2% protein, and 15% water[7], and since the energy values of these components are approximately 9, 4 and 0 kcal/g respectively, it follows that the energy value of 1 kg of adipose tissue is about 7550 kcal/kg. As a first approximation we may think of lean body mass as 25% protein and 75% water, and the glycogen – water pool as 25% glycogen and 75% water[8]. This gives a convenient value of 1000 kcal/kg for both lean body mass and the glycogen – water pool.

If this quantitative model is applied to the problem of a middle-aged woman on a diet supplying 1000 kcal per day, it is possible to reconcile differences in rate of weight loss. If she is actually keeping strictly to the prescribed diet, and has a total energy expenditure of 2000 kcal per day, the deficit of 1000 kcal daily must be met by sacrifice of some part of the energy stores of her body. If she is burning exclusively adipose tissue the expected rate of weight loss would be about 1 kg per week, since this is an energy store of about 7000 kcal. However if she was starting on a reducing diet with replete stores of glycogen she might well burn 3·5 kg of glycogen – water mixture and only 0·5 kg of adipose tissue in the first week. This is the same 7000 kcal debit to the energy stores, but it would be reflected in a weight loss of 4 kg instead of 1 kg.

The second type of problem encountered by obese patients is that despite their best endeavours they lose no weight at all. If body weight has not changed the explanation must be either that energy intake has matched energy output, so no weight change is to be expected, or alternatively that a decrease in adipose tissue has been masked by a compensatory increase in some other component of body weight, such as water. The latter may explain short-term fluctuations in body weight (say up to 1 kg over periods of a few days[9]) but is unlikely to explain large discrepancies in weight loss, unless there is some very obvious disorder of regulation of body water, or if normal regulation of water has been upset by injudicious use of diuretics.

In practice a rate of weight loss of less than 0·5 kg (1 lb) per week is usually unsatisfactory: if a patient needs to lose 25 kg this should be achieved within 1 year. From the calculation given above about the energy value of adipose tissue a loss of 0·5 kg per week of adipose tissue represents an energy loss of about 500 kcal per day from the body stores. To state the proposition the other way round, anyone who fails to lose 0·5 kg per week on average over a period of many weeks must have an energy intake which is less than 500 kcal per day below energy expenditure. This situation often arises when the patient is not given good dietary advice, or does not follow the advice accurately. Consider the advice given in a recent booklet issued by the Health Educational Council[10]: 'If you are more than 2 stone overweight you can safely increase your calorie allowance to 1500 for women. . . . If you follow the eating plan conscientiously you should lose an average of 2–3 lb per week.' This is misleading advice. There are obese women in whom total energy expenditure is about 2000 kcal daily, so if such patients accurately maintain an intake of 1500 kcal daily it is not to be expected that they will continue to lose more than 0·5 kg (1 lb) per week.

It is also fair to say that relatively few patients who aim to take 1500 kcal per day actually achieve this objective every day. When outpatients, who have failed to lose weight on a prescribed diet, are admitted to a closely controlled metabolic ward and fed exactly the same diet, they usually lose weight. This observation has led many practitioners to take an unduly cynical view of 'cheating' on reducing diets, so that failure to lose weight is regarded as proof of deviation from the diet. Thus Jolliffe and Alpert[11] devised a formula by which they thought that they could predict the rate at which patients should lose weight: 'It is on this basis that we categorically accuse each subject of dietary errors whenever they fail to equal at least 85% of prediction. Whenever they do better than 115% of prediction we tell them that they are losing excess fluid.' The arrogance of this attitude is breathtaking, since it does not require a very penetrating analysis to show that the 'error' of 15% is at least as likely to lie in the prediction formula as in the patient's eating habits[7].

The third category of patients complain that they simply cannot keep to the diet. They agree that a weight loss of a pound a week or so would be quite reasonable; they agree that if they actually kept to the prescribed diet they would lose weight at this rate; they agree that they really want and need to lose weight and do not expect any magic cure which contravenes the laws of thermodynamics; but having agreed all that, they still say that the effort of dieting is more than they can manage. They may well volunteer the diagnosis that they are 'compulsive eaters'.

In some cases the patient's analysis is quite correct, and the effort of trying to lose weight is too great for the benefit which this would bring. This aspect is considered under the next heading on the cost and benefit of weight loss. However it is relevant to the question of expectation and motivation to define more closely the diagnosis of a 'compulsive eater'. Sometimes this phrase is used in letters referring patients to a hospital clinic, when the patient's attitude to food is absolutely normal. Anyone who has tried to alter his diet for several weeks in some important respect knows that it is irksome. Even if the food is perfectly palatable and adequate to satisfy hunger it is very irritating to have to remember not to eat certain items if, for example, you are on a purine-free diet. If the diet is designed to be deficient in energy (as all reducing diets are) it is still less pleasant since, in addition to the general constraint of eating what is prescribed rather than what you fancy, there is the added stimulus of hunger. It is not surprising that most patients find it difficult to keep to a reducing diet, but this certainly does not make them compulsive eaters. People vary in their drive to eat, and those who attend obesity clinics may be selected for a greater-than-average drive to eat. Within this population there are some who are indeed compulsive eaters. They may describe eating behaviour which is totally unrelated to hunger: they may have eating binges which are ultimately limited only by nausea or stupor, and which go on for days at a time. This is a condition which should be clearly distinguished from the difficulties and lapses which any normal person will have when trying to follow a reducing diet.

The three main categories of motivation and expectation in patients trying to lose weight have been outlined above. The other important factor in prognosis is the motivation and expectation of the doctor. Because most obese patients seeking medical advice will have already tried to lose weight and failed, it is naive to suppose that a diet sheet passed across the consulting-room table will be a passport to success. In an average general practice there will be about 40 patients with severe and long-standing obesity[12]. To treat these patients requires a considerable investment of time and determination by the practitioner. Other patients with relatively trivial obesity will also compete for his attention. It is therefore necessary to choose between treating everyone inadequately, or selecting a few who can be treated well. The second course is preferable. It has been suggested that one of the criteria for selecting obese patients for treatment is that they should not have failed to lose weight in the past[13]. This proposal is difficult to justify[7], but if other practitioners apply it then there is a grave responsibility on anyone starting to treat a severely obese patient that the treatment should not unnecessarily fail. This may discourage not only the patient, but also other doctors who might otherwise have tried to help.

COST *VERSUS* BENEFIT IN WEIGHT LOSS

It is unfortunate that in weight loss the cost, in terms of inconvenience both
to patient and doctor, is immediately obvious, while the benefits resulting
from weight loss are more distant and hence less obvious. In some diseases,
such as gluten-sensitive enteropathy, it may be expected that there will be
a marked change in the patient's health within a few weeks of starting the
therapeutic diet, but with obesity the rewards (if any) are not seen for
months or years. Therefore gluten-sensitive patients usually are more
vigilant to maintain their gluten-free diet than obese patients are to maintain a low energy intake. Indeed there are many patients trying to lose
weight in whom it would be unreasonable to suggest that the rewards were
worth the struggle.

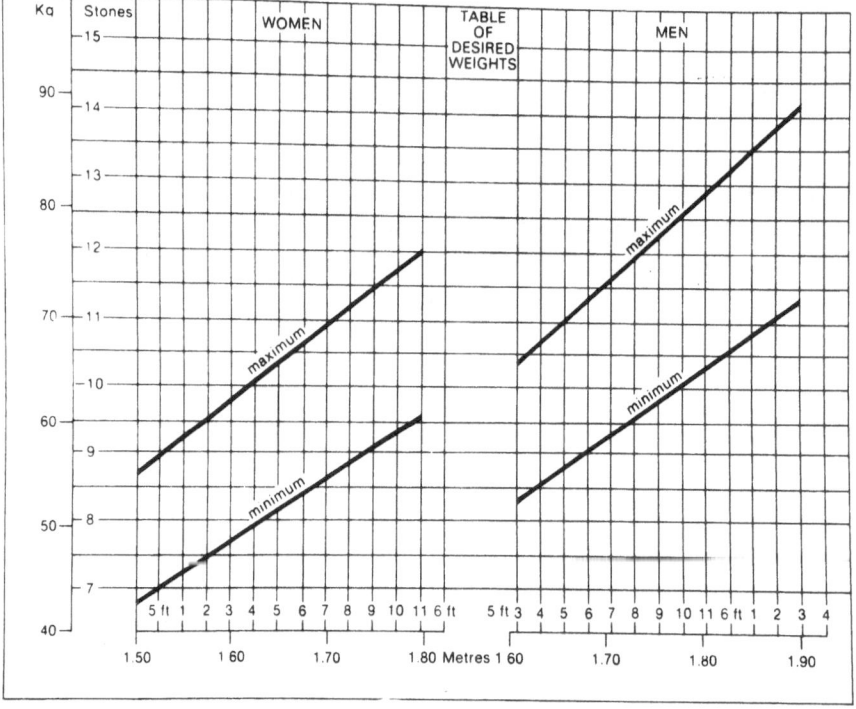

Figure 1 Range of desirable weight-for-height in men and women, based on life
insurance mortality experience. Weight is measured in indoor clothing, and height
without shoes

It is convenient to use the chart shown in Figure 1 to classify patients
into those who are, or are not, likely to benefit from weight loss. The lines

marking the maximum and minimum limits of 'desirable' weight for height for women and men are based on the experience of the Metropolitan Life Assurance Company and encompass the maximum of the 'large frame' to the minimum of the 'small frame'. Probably it was a mistake to introduce the concept of frame size into these charts at all, since there is no agreed way of measuring frame size. For those who prefer to carry pocket calculators rather than copies of Figure 1 much the same criteria of desirable weight can be obtained by using the ratio of W/H^2, where W is weight in kg and H height in metres. For women the maximum desirable weight line corresponds to a W/H^2 of about 24·2, and for men about 25·0. (For those who measure in pounds and inches, the corresponding ratios would be 0·035 and 0·036 respectively.) The chart form has the great advantage that patients are able to recognize their weight in relation to the desirable range. This is useful when adolescents (or their parents) are unduly worried about their fatness or thinness: if in fact they are within the normal range there is no medical indication for weight change, but there may still be cosmetic reasons which are outside the scope of this chapter.

The association between overweight and mortality has been well summarized by Donald[14]: at all ages and in both sexes overweight is associated with increased rates of mortality. The causes of death reported more often in overweight than normal weight subjects are diabetes, cardiovascular and renal disease, and disease of the biliary tract. An important cause of morbidity associated with obesity is osteoarthritis of the weight-bearing joints[15], and childbirth, surgery and anaesthesia are more dangerous and difficult in obese patients than thin ones[7]. Recent prospective studies have found little evidence of an association between obesity and coronary heart disease when factors such as age, blood pressure, smoking and serum cholesterol were taken into account[16], and this finding has been interpreted to mean that the observed coronary mortality in obese people is a coincidence rather than a causal relationship, so obesity in itself is a benign condition. This is poor reasoning. Among 11 400 men aged 40–59 at entry to the study[16] there were 217 who had heart attacks within the next 5 years. If they are divided into fat and thin on the basis of skinfolds 1·60% of thin men, and 2·67% of fat men had heart attacks. The age-group chosen for the study is one in which heart attacks are common, but the effect of obesity on mortality is relatively small. Table 1 is taken from the study by Blair and Haines[17] on the mortality experience of men who passed a medical examination for life insurance at normal rates. This shows that the association between overweight and increased mortality is strongest among young men (aged 15–34 at examination) and that the excess mortality peaks at 21–25 years after insurance: that is, when these men are in their 40s and 50s. In the age-group studied by Keys and his colleagues[16] the association between overweight and mortality is relatively small.

Table 1 Percentage of average mortality in men who passed a medical examination for life insurance, and duration of policy at death (data from Blair and Haines, 1966[17])

Age at issue (years)	Deviation from standard weight	Policy years				All policies
		16–20	21–25	26–30	31–34	
15–34	− 23 lb or more	102	78	80	95	86
	− 22 to − 8 lb	77	76	91	98	86
	− 7 to + 7 lb	82	107	108	108	103
	+ 8 to + 22 lb	166	131	115	94	125
	+ 23 lb or more	137	184	143	—	146
35–49	− 23 lb or more	67	84	86	72	80
	− 22 to − 8 lb	79	83	77	84	80
	− 7 to + 7 lb	104	91	105	86	99
	+ 8 to + 22 lb	116	117	108	119	115
	+ 23 lb or more	119	134	132	169	130
50–65	− 23 lb or more	—	—	120	—	95
	− 22 to − 8 lb	97	108	102	—	100
	− 7 to + 7 lb	98	87	81	88	90
	+ 8 to + 22 lb	109	102	113	—	108
	+ 23 lb or more	107	125	122	—	118

The second piece of evidence that obesity is not benign is the finding that people who are refused insurance at normal premiums because they are overweight, but who then reduce to the 'desirable range', subsequently enjoy normal mortality experience. This is based on a review of 2300 people, and Dublin[18] observes: 'A test of this kind is about as objective as one could ask.'

There is a third factor which may also explain the difference between the strong association found by life insurance companies between over-weight and mortality, and the relatively weak association found in some, but not all, prospective epidemiological surveys. Epidemiologists arrange thorough routine examination of the subjects they are studying, whether or not these subjects are complaining of ill-health. In real life, in order to be thoroughly examined, a patient has to convince a doctor that there is some illness worth looking for, and this is a more difficult task for a fat patient than a thin one. If a thin person complains of tiredness, change in bowel habit, shortness of breath, or muscle or joint pain, it is likely that a doctor will first consider the numerous diseases of which these may be the pre-senting symptoms, and investigate accordingly. However a fat patient with the identical symptoms (and therefore the same chance of having the same diseases) may well be told that these symptoms are the consequence of obesity, or the diet or medicine which has been prescribed for the obesity, and the approptiate investigations are delayed, or never undertaken. Even if the doctor does try to exclude other diseases, all diagnostic procedures, from physical examination to radiography, are more difficult to do well in fat people. One of the undocumented hazards of obesity is that the over-weight patient is likely to receive a lower standard of medical care[19].

Thus it is possible to state with some confidence the medical benefits from weight loss which can be expected by a young person who is, say, 10 kg or more above the maximum of the desirable weight for height. Briefly these are improved exercise tolerance, increased life expectancy by avoiding diabetes and ischaemic heart disease, less morbidity by avoiding osteoarthritis of weight-bearing joints and gall-bladder disease, and less trouble and danger if and when they need an anaesthetic or surgical operation. The greater the degree of overweight the more true these state-ments become. In older patients the hazards of overweight still exist, but the chance of avoiding them by weight loss are less for two reasons: first, with increasing age metabolic rate decreases, so it is more difficult to generate the energy deficit on which weight loss depends; and second, even if old people do achieve significant weight loss the damage done by over-weight is only partly reversible.

Patients who seek psychological or social benefits from weight loss are involved in a more speculative investment. In some grossly overweight young people the motivation for weight loss is entirely social: they are not yet disabled, and are not at all concerned with the long-term medical disadvantages of obesity. They may be intensely concerned to lose weight in the expectation that this would bring social acceptability, and often fall prey to charlatans who promise rapid effortless weight loss as a solution to their problems. These people require help, since if they continue to seek magic cures they are likely to become demoralized as well as financially impoverished. If such patients can be persuaded to adopt a realistic attitude about the rate of weight loss which can be achieved, and the benefits which this is likely to bring, the doctor will have performed a valuable service. In fact there often are great psychological and social benefits following weight loss, but sometimes there is depressingly little gain in this respect. At present it is not possible to distinguish in advance between the patient in whom obesity is a prime cause of unhappiness, and one who would be just as unhappy after weight loss. One can only try, and see.

The cost of weight loss was eloquently described by a patient addressing his physician in 1825[1]: 'Sir, I have followed your prescription as if my life depended upon it, and I have ascertained that during this month I have lost three pounds or a little more. But in order to reach this result I have been obliged to do such violence to all my tastes and all my habits – in a word I have suffered so much – that while giving you my best thanks for your kind directions, I renounce any advantages from them and throw myself for the future entirely into the hands of Providence.' No patient should be expected to suffer so much for a loss of three pounds in a month, unless it can be shown that still greater suffering would be incurred by *not* losing three pounds in a month, and this is rarely the case.

The problem, therefore, is to find a line of treatment which causes an energy deficit of at least 500 kcal per day, and which does the least violence to the patient's tastes and habits. Obviously if these habits include consuming 10 pints of beer each evening the habits will have to change or little weight loss will be achieved, so the problem then is one of convincing the patient that the potential gain is greater than the required sacrifice. The best option for a given patient often emerges after several visits to the doctor. There will be many problems which are not evident on the first occasion when the patient is given dietary advice: the difficulties become clear when an attempt is made to put the advice into practice. It saves time to enquire what difficulties prevented the patient from following dietary advice in the past, since these can be forestalled. For example if the patient attends social functions which are incompatible with a reducing diet it is necessary to decide if higher priority should be given to weight loss or to attending the social functions. If the patient's spouse insists that the standard of catering in the home should not be affected by the patient's effort at dieting, it should be established that the spouse realizes that the choice is between altering the menus or having the wife/husband disabled to an extent that, instead of contributing to the running of the household, they would themselves require looking after. If these points can fairly be made, many patients who previously found dieting 'impossible' come to regard it as the least of available evils.

INVOLVEMENT OF A THIRD PARTY IN THERAPY

Even the most conscientious doctor is unlikely to spend more than a few minutes per week with an obese patient discussing the problems of treatment, so for the great majority of the time the motivation to persist must come from some other source. One of the great merits of slimming groups is that they provide mutual support and encouragement, but the patient who has lapsed from treatment may well cease to attend the doctor or slimming group. It is necessary, therefore, to strike a balance between providing constant policing of the obese patient, and a reasonable respect for individual liberty. The involvement of a third party, such as the spouse of the patient, may either help or hinder treatment, depending on the attitude of the people involved.

An excellent example of an unhelpful third party is the anxious mother of a fat adolescent. It requires more tact than most parents can muster to help teenage offspring with any problem at all, and a subject so delicate as diet is particularly likely to provoke mutiny rather than cooperation. Among sensible adults, however, it is often possible to set up constructive alliances which will help and encourage a dieting patient. The husband who promises some lavish bribe for substantial weight loss by his wife is not particularly helpful, since these arrangements tend to turn sour whether the target is, or is not, achieved. It is more constructive if the spouse (or other member of the family) takes care not to make dieting more difficult by having particularly attractive food in evidence, keeps a watch on the actual weight loss achieved, and encourages the patient to attend the doctor or slimming club. In all these arrangements it is essential that the policy is agreed beforehand, and seen to benefit both parties in the long run. Punitive measures imposed by one member of the family on another have little chance of success in maintaining weight loss. However one woman has arranged with her husband that her use of the family car is contingent on maintaining a loss of at least 1 pound per week. This system seems to work very well: her weight loss is comfortably ahead of this minimum rate, and she says that on the occasions when in the past she would have had an eating binge she has refrained, since the inconvenience of being without transport deters her.

All such schemes are not a substitute for primary motivation: the patient has to be convinced that an analysis of the cost and benefit of weight loss, as set out above, shows that the effort in the long term is worth while. The best that can be expected of domestically arranged incentive schemes is that the benefit of refraining from an eating binge is made immediate (e.g. use of family car) rather than distant.

WHEN TO TREAT: PROBLEMS SPECIFIC TO AGE GROUPS

Infancy
The hypothesis 'that obesity may be accompanied by an excessive number of adipocytes, possibly brought about by excess feeding in infancy and childhood, and that the excessive number of adipocytes remains constant and in some way causes a drive for maintaining the obese state', was advanced by Hirsch[20]. It is true that very obese patients have more fat cells, detectable by current laboratory methods, than slightly obese patients, and it is also often true that very obese patients become fat early in life. However the hypothesis set out above has not been established by further investigation. When patients with the same amount of fat are compared there is no significant relationship between the age of onset of obesity and the number of fat cells[21,22]. Thus it is no longer likely that infancy is a

'critical period' at which feeding practices predestine the child to obesity, or confer lifelong immunity from it. It is still reasonable not to overfeed babies, and not to misinterpret thirst as hunger, but recent follow-up studies show that in general fat babies do not remain fat[23]. I would not give high priority to *treating* obesity in infancy, but would take reasonable care to prevent it developing.

The primary school child

Between the ages of about 5 and 12 years there is an opportunity for treating obesity which should not be missed. The child is growing fairly quickly, so if the gain in weight can be held to a lower rate than the gain in height the weight : height ratio will improve without having to achieve any actual weight loss. The definition of obesity at this age should be based on skinfold thickness: the sum of the triceps and subscapular skinfolds exceeds 30 mm in about 6% of children at this age[24], and these children should receive special attention from the school medical service. If they then enter secondary school with a normal amount of body fat this may save much trouble later.

Adolescence

The period from age 13 to 16 is a particularly unrewarding one for the treatment of obesity. The adolescent child who is brought to the doctor for treatment of obesity is obviously not particularly willing or able to lose weight. The arguments which have been advanced above as benefits from weight loss will make little impact on such a child, and I cannot think of a patient in this age-range to whom my advice has been any use. We might as well declare this a closed season for the treatment of obesity. By the age of 17 the young adult may decide to assume responsibility for control of his or her body weight, and at that stage it is possible to commence treatment with reasonable prospects of success.

Pregnancy

Obstetric fashions vary: some obstetricians argue that since feeding a sow lavishly produces big piglets a similar policy should be applied to pregnant women[25]. It is true that in women of normal weight there is a correlation between the mother's weight gain and the size of the baby, but this relationship does not hold for women who are overweight before starting the pregnancy. There is no reason why an obese woman should not provide the 200 kcal per day, which is the energy cost of a normal pregnancy[26], from her excess fat stores, rather than eating enough to maintain both her pregnancy and her obesity. The available evidence shows that the fetus is an efficient parasite, and in the human species (unlike farm animals) a moderate degree of dietary reduction in an obese mother does nothing to impair fetal growth. Analysis of the development of children born during the severe famine in Holland in the winter of 1944–45 has failed to show any mental or physical impairment[27]. It is important that pregnancy should *not* be regarded as a closed season for the treatment of obesity. Pregnancy is a time when women are susceptible to dietary advice, and this is an opportunity to prevent the development of obesity in the mother, and perhaps in her child also.

Lactation
It is hard to find reliable evidence about the effects of moderate dietary restriction of lactating women, but in principle it seems unwise to reduce energy intake at a time when the mother has an increased energy output in breast milk which is much greater than the increased energy cost of pregnancy. Many mothers do not breast-feed for long, but they should be encouraged to do so, and dietary restriction should not be made a cause, or an excuse, to give up suckling.

Old age
Obesity is common in old age, and difficult to treat. If the function of a doctor is to make life more tolerable for the patient, this objective is often unattainable to any useful degree by restricting the food intake of old people.

CHOOSING THE BEST TREATMENT FOR THE PATIENT

There is no consensus about the 'best' treatment for obesity, nor is a treatment which is appropriate for one patient necessarily suitable for another. My own practice is to proceed in a series of steps, with the hope of finding a line of treatment which is effective in producing fat loss without too much loss of lean tissue, which is acceptable to the patient, and unlikely to do harm.

The first step is to establish if the patient is likely to benefit from weight loss, and if so what steps have been taken to achieve this in the past, and why they have failed. If the patient has never tried a properly constructed reducing diet, with a realistic assessment of the weight loss which this is likely to produce[28], then this is the obvious first step.

If this is tried for a month or so and fails, it must be either because the requirements of the patient are so low that the reducing diet did not generate the expected energy deficit, or alternatively that the patient did not follow the diet. The correct explanation may be discovered by asking the patient, or it may be necessary to undertake inpatient investigations to establish the patient's metabolic rate and body composition, and what in fact happens when the prescribed diet is fed under controlled conditions[7]. If the patient's metabolic rate is low the obvious therapy is to use a thermogenic drug, but the hazards of this line of treatment are usually greater than that of the obesity itself. If the patient's metabolic rate is normal, and fat is lost at the expected rate on the prescribed diet, the problem is one of assisting the patient to keep to the diet.

In some cases the patient, having observed that weight loss was indeed achieved at the predicted rate on the prescribed diet, is encouraged to try harder to keep to the diet. However some very obese patients cannot contemplate the possibility of years of self-denial to achieve massive weight loss, and in these some form of surgery may be useful. The best policy we have tried is wiring the jaws for about 9 months to achieve weight loss, and following this with a gastric bypass operation if necessary to prevent weight gain after the wires are removed. Other lines of treatment are presented elsewhere in this book.

PREVENTION OF OBESITY

It would be very desirable to prevent obesity, but there are great difficulties in achieving this objective. Even if it were possible and acceptable to ensure that each person, each day, had an energy intake from food which was exactly the amount recommended by various government committees, this policy would not prevent obesity. The best a committee can do is to estimate that (for example) a woman between the age of 18 and 55 years who weighs 55 kg, requires on average 2200 kcal per day. However some of these women will use 1900 kcal, and some 2500 kcal per day, so if they were all fed the same ration some would be about 100 000 kcal in positive balance by the end of the year (i.e. would have gained about 14 kg of adipose tissue), while others would be well on the way to emaciation. This range of individual variation in energy requirements is far larger than the error in energy balance required to cause rapidly developing obesity, so no prevention scheme based on a rationing system is likely to work.

Some health education workers seem to believe that there are specific foods which are particularly liable to lead to obesity. So there may be for individuals, but taste as well as metabolism varies from person to person, so it would be quite misguided to ban certain foodstuffs in the hope of preventing obesity. It would not have the desired effect, and would unnecessarily deprive the rest of the population of an acceptable food.

If it were possible to predict a section of the population who were particularly prone to obesity a prevention programme might be based on a careful monitoring of the weight gain in this group. Unfortunately attempts at identifying such a group have not been successful. For example an analysis of the pattern of weight gain of children in infancy fails to reveal which of them will be overweight at age 7 years[29]. Among children who are overweight at age 10 years about half were already overweight at age 5 years, but retrospective examination of the weight curve of those who were of normal weight at 5 years does not show any characteristics which would differentiate between these children and those who were normal weight at 5 years and continued to be normal weight at 10 years[30].

In practice the nearest practical approach to prevention is early treatment. This also presents difficulties, because it is undesirable to make an entire poulation anxious about possible weight gain. Indeed it may be argued that publicity along these lines would do more harm by precipitating anorexia nervosa than the good it would do in limiting minor degrees of obesity. However the range of weight shown in Figure 1 is wide, and if it is established that there is no special merit in being at the middle, or lower edge, of this range, it should serve as a reminder to people who are crossing the maximum line that they are overweight. The sooner this is noticed the sooner some action is likely to be taken, and hence the more likely it is that they will be able to make a fairly painless descent into the normal range again. I am not suggesting that doctors should immediately assume responsibility for anyone who crosses the maximum line, since on this policy the National Health Service would soon be overwhelmed. I believe this is a group of moderately obese patients for whom slimming clubs may be the best form of treatment.

SUMMARY

The treatment of severe obesity is a slow and difficult business both for doctor and patient, so the doctor should concentrate upon the patients who will benefit most from weight loss. In general these are the youngest and the most overweight. These patients need a realistic assessment of the advantages of weight loss, and what the cost is likely to be. Half-hearted treatment is worse than useless. Failed treatment converts obese patients into 'refractory' obese patients, so before starting treatment the doctor should consider if he can give the necessary time and attention to the problem.

The objective is to create a negative energy balance, such that the patient will lose adipose tissue without too great a loss of lean tissue, in a manner which is as acceptable as possible to the patient, and which is unlikely to do harm. In practice a rate of weight loss between 1 and 2 lb (0·5–1·0 kg) per week is usually best in the long run for outpatients, but individual patients will have very different requirements to achieve this rate of weight loss.

Most obese patients attending the doctor will have already tried, and failed, to lose weight elsewhere. It is necessary to find out what treatment has already been tried, and why it failed, if the same mistakes are not to be repeated.

It is difficult to prevent obesity. The best policy is to inform the public that those whose weight exceeds the maximum of the desirable range of weight for height are probably incurring medical hazards. The sooner people in this situation take the appropriate action the more likely they are to regain the normal weight range, and the less trouble this will be.

References

1 Astwood, E. B. (1962). The heritage of corpulence. *Endocrinology*, **71**, 337
2 Kemp, R. (1972). The overall picture of obesity. *Practitioner*, **209**, 654
3 Goldrick, R. B., Havenstein, N. and Whyte, H. M. (1973). Effect of caloric restriction and fenfluramine on weight loss and personality profile of patients with longstanding obesity. *Aust. N.Z. J. Med.*, **3**, 131
4 Garrow, J. S. (1976). Upbringing, appetite and adult obesity. In A. W. Wilkinson (ed.). *Early Nutrition and Later Development*, pp. 219–228. (London: Pitman Medical Publ.)
5 Ashwell, M. A. (1973). A survey investigating patients' views on doctors' treatment of obesity. *Practitioner*, **211**, 653
6 Dwyer, J. T. and Mayer, J. (1970). Potential dieters: who are they? Attitudes towards body weight and dieting behaviour. *J. Am. Diet. Assoc.*, **56**, 510
7 Garrow, J. S. (1978). *Energy Balance and Obesity in Man*, 2nd edn. (Amsterdam: North Holland Publishing Co.)
8 Olsson, E.-E. and Saltin, B. (1970). Variation in total body water with muscle glycogen in man. *Acta Physiol. Scand.*, **80**, 11
9 Edholm, O. G., Adam, J. M. and Best, T. W. (1974). Day-to-day weight changes in young men. *Ann. Hum. Biol.*, **1**, 3
10 MacAdie, D. (1978). *Eat your way to better health*. (London: Health Education Council)
11 Jolliffe, N. and Alpert, E. (1951). The 'performance index' as a method for estimating effectiveness of reducing regimens. *Postgrad. Med.*, **9**, 106
12 Binnie, C. C. (1977). Obesity in general practice. Ten year follow-up of obesity. *J. Roy. Coll. Gen. Pract.*, **27**, 492
13 Young, C. M. (1963). Management of the obese patient. *J. Am. Med. Assoc.*, **186**, 903
14 Donald, D. W. A. (1973). Mortality rates among the overweight. In R. F. Robertson (ed.), *Anorexia and Obesity*, pp. 63–70. (Edinburgh: RCP)
15 Leach, R. E., Baumgard, S. and Broom, J. (1973). Obesity: its relationship to osteoarthritis of the knee. *Clin. Orthop.*, **93**, 271
16 Keys, A., Aravanis, C., Blackburn, H., Buchem, F. S. P., Buzina, R., Djordjevic, B. S., Fidansa, F., Karvonen, M. J., Menotti, V. and Taylor, H. L. (1972). Coronary heart disease: overweight and obesity as risk factors. *Ann. Intern. Med.*, **77**, 15
17 Blair, B. F. and Haines, L. W. (1966). Mortality experience according to build at higher durations. *Trans. Act. Soc. Amer.*, **18**, 35
18 Dublin, L. I. (1953). Relation of obesity to longevity. *N. Engl. J. Med.*, **248**, 971

19 Garrow, J. S. (1976). Underfeeding and overfeeding and their clinical consequences. *Proc. Nutr. Soc.*, **35,** 363

20 Hirsch, J. (1974). Cell number and size as a determinant of subsequent obesity. In M. Winick (ed.) *Childhood Obesity*, pp. 15–21. (New York: Wiley)

21 Hirsch, J. and Batchelor, B. (1976). Adipose tissue cellularity in human obesity. *Clin. Endocr. Metab.*, **5,** 299

22 Ashwell, M. A., Durrant, M. and Garrow, J. S. (1977). How a 'fat cell pool' hypothesis could account for the relationship between adipose tissue cellularity and age of onset of obesity. *Proc. Nutr. Soc.*, **36,** 111A

23 Poskitt, E. M. E. and Cole, T. J. (1977). Do fat babies stay fat? *Br. Med. J.*, **1,** 7

24 Whitelaw, A. G. J. (1971). The association of social class and sibling number with skinfold thickness in London schoolboys. *Hum. Biol.*, **43,** 414

25 Brewer, T. (1967). Human pregnancy nutrition: a clinical view. *Obstet. Gynecol.*, **30,** 605

26 Blackburn, N. W. and Calloway, D. H. (1976). Energy expenditure and consumption of mature, pregnant and lactating women. *J. Am. Diet. Assoc.*, **69,** 29

27 Stein, Z., Susser, M., Saenger, G., and Marolla, F. (1975). *Famine and Human Development: the Dutch Hunger Winter of 1944–1945*, p. 284. (London: Oxford University Press)

28 Ford, M. J., Scorgie, R. E. and Munro, J. F. (1977). Anticipated rate of weight loss during dieting. *Int. J. Obesity*, **1,** 239

29 Mellbin, T. and Vuille, J.-C. (1973). Physical development at 7 years in relation to velocity of weight gain in infancy with special reference to incidence of overweight. *Br. J. Brev. Soc. Med.*, **27,** 225

30 Wilkinson, P. W., Parkin, J. M., Pearlson, J., Philips, P. R. and Sykes, P. (1977). Obesity in childhood: a community study in Newcastle upon Tyne. *Lancet*, **i,** 350

2

Dietary management of obesity and obesity-related diseases

A. C. MacCuish and M. J. Ford

INTRODUCTION

Obesity is the commonest nutritional disorder in the Western world. If defined as a body weight in excess of 20% of desirable weight, it affects 20% of men and 30% of women[1]. Many will make strenuous attempts to cure themselves before seeking medical advice, though the number who succeed remains unknown. From the Consumers' Association question-naire, 42% of over 2000 people who had previously attempted to lose weight had never sought medical advice[2] and in a survey of obese subjects attending a Slimming Club, 80% had previously tried to lose weight on their own[3].

It is therefore not surprising that those patients whose obesity does not respond readily to self-imposed dietary restriction often comprise the groups of 'refractory' obese who consult their general or hospital practitioner and in whom the results of therapy are generally so poor.

Management aims

Since the majority of obese patients seeking medical advice for the first time will have tried to lose weight previously, it follows that a degree of good intent will be present and their request for assistance must be taken seriously. The first steps in management should be to identify those problems which are judged to cause, underlie or accompany the complaint of obesity and to recognize that associated and often more important pathological factors (psychological stress, cigarette-smoking, hypertension, diabetes and hyperlipoproteinaemia) may be present. The aims of therapy should be to deepen the patient's understanding of his own weight problem and achieve a satisfactory weight loss by a change in eating behaviour. For some patients it will soon become clear that it may be better to help them adapt to, and accept, their weight problem and to focus attention on other associated factors. For others, the aim may be transient weight loss and once this has served its purpose, e.g. enabling a surgical operation or attendance at a social function, they may elect to return to their previous eating habit. However, the majority will require to change their eating pattern permanently, adopt a realistic concept of the anticipated rate of weight loss and remain appropriately motivated if therapy is to have any lasting success[4].

The approach
The establishment of a satisfactory rapport with the patient is always essential and requires a combination of skill, empathy and tact. Various studies have shown that the quality of the therapist, repeated consultation with the same therapist and regular long-term follow-up are all important factors determining success[5-7]. The first interview with the obese must include an assessment of the degree of motivation to lose weight and identification of the major stimulus which precipitated the decision to seek medical advice. The Consumers' Association survey found that a majority of women wanted to lose weight in order to improve their appearance while most men wanted to lose weight for health reasons[8]. While it is self-evident that the highly motivated will be more successful, other predictive factors of success include the degree of insight into the origin of obesity, the patient's level of social conformity and the desire for social acceptance[9]. Silverstone and Solomon showed that the non-neurotic obese fared better than the neurotic[10]. Others have shown that the co-existence of physical illness, e.g. hypertension, has a favourable influence on the outcome of attempted weight reduction[11,12] though this does not seem true of diabetes mellitus[13]. Many people have grossly unrealistic concepts of the rate of weight loss to be expected after starting a diet, and when they fail to achieve such a rate, may become disheartened and abandon their attempts to reduce, whilst in fact making satisfactory progress[3]. Every effort should be made to establish and reinforce realistic concepts of the rate of anticipated weight loss. Naturally, weight loss cannot exceed about 2 lb (1 kg) per week given a daily energy deficit of 1000 kcal (4·2 MJ) after the first two weeks of dieting. In this respect, it is important to discourage the common practice of daily weighing and to advise patients to weigh themselves on the same scales, in the same clothing, not more than once every fortnight. Since weight loss is progressive, albeit slow, the final target weight will usually take some months to achieve. Again, this time-scale should be emphasized to the patient to strengthen the concept that dieting really does mean a different way of life if the target weight is to be achieved

and maintained. Unless the figure is absurdly low or high, it is seldom necessary to correct the patient's own idea of target weight, especially since the excess cardiovascular risk of obesity is minimal in individuals less than 30% overweight[14].

The next step is to document the pattern of eating behaviour which has led to obesity, and to identify any obvious stresses which precipitate inappropriate eating. It is axiomatic that all the overweight have consumed an energy intake in excess of their requirements at some time but few obese patients consistently over-eat. In the minority, a high intake of one or two specific carbohydrate sources will be found to have caused the weight problem. More usually, it will be necessary to isolate those characteristics of life-style and eating behaviour which have culminated in the achievement and perpetuation of obesity. A record should be made of the patient's eating pattern, including meal frequency and content, and activities and feelings at the time of eating. In this way, a considerable degree of insight may be gained, both by the patient and physician, which permits modification of subsequent eating behaviour and isolates unintentional or inadvertent sources of caloric intake.

At the conclusion of the interview, and before detailed dietary advice is given, a search should be made for associated health problems, by physical examination. This will normally include a clinical assessment of thyroid and cardiac status and the analysis of urine for the presence of glucose and protein. Where appropriate, a glucose tolerance test and fasting plasma lipid screen should also be performed.

THE DIET IN SIMPLE OBESITY

General considerations

The success of dietary treatment for obesity is directly related to the ease with which a new and permanent eating pattern is adopted. It follows that the principal aim of any diet in the management of simple obesity is that the diet should immediately reduce food intake and yet be potentially permanent. With this aim in view, only those diets considered suitable for a permanent way of life are considered here.

If a satisfactory rate of weight loss (1–2 lb or $\frac{1}{2}$–1 kg per week) is to be achieved, then the diet selected should produce a daily energy deficit of 500–1000 kcal (2·1–4·2 MJ). The optimum reducing regimen in adults should reduce calorie intake by approximately 50%, falling within the range of 800-1500 kcal per day (3·3–6·3 MJ) and it should be remembered that the daily energy requirements may vary enormously from one individual to the next, as well as being considerably influenced by age and sex (Table 1)[15].

Table 1   Recommended normal daily energy requirements[15] (NB: in adults this may vary from 1500 to 5000 kcal daily)

Population and age (years)	Daily energy requirements (kcal)
CHILDREN	
1	800
1–2	1200
2–3	1400
3–5	1600
5–7	1800
7–9	2100
FEMALES	
9–18	2300
18–55	2200–2500
(55 kg) 55–75	2050
75+	1900
Pregnancy	2400 (2nd and 3rd trimester)
Lactation	2700
MALES	
9–12	2500
12–15	2800
15–18	3000
(65 kg) 18–35	2700–3600
35–65	2600–3600
65–76	2350
75+	2100

1000 kcal = 4·2 MJ; 1 MJ = 240 kcal

(Data from Dept. of Health and Social Security (1969), *Reports on Public Health and Medical Subjects*, No. 120 (HMSO))

Diets in obesity – needs and wants
Any reducing regimen selected to become a way of life must provide a suitable energy deficit together with essential nutrients and additionally, should be simple, satisfying, palatable, inexpensive and socially acceptable. A number of other factors may also be relevant to the optimal diet; these may exert subtle but significant effects on calorie intake and include meal frequency, caloric density of foodstuffs and fibre intake.

Meal frequency
Studies in animals and man have established that the timing of food intake may have important metabolic effects. Obese subjects often eat irregularly, taking two-thirds of their calorie intake after mid-day, compared with the non-obese who consume two-thirds of their calorie intake before noon.

Since the synthesis rates of protein are subject to a diurnal variation which may be related to the rhythm of cortisol secretion, it has been proposed that meals taken before mid-day and in the late evening may be utilised more efficiently than meals taken at other times[16]. Fabry and his colleagues showed that men who ate more than three meals per day had a lower incidence of obesity, hypercholesterolaemia and impaired glucose tolerance than those who ate less frequently[17]. However, in clinical practice, weight loss is comparable in obese patients eating 1000 kcal (4·2 MJ) daily whether this intake is divided between two or five meals[18,19]. Patient compliance is often better using a two-meal-per-day regimen, though some find a multi-meal plan more successful in suppressing appetite and promoting weight loss.

Calorie density
The response of obese subjects to caloric dilution is difficult to interpret and different from that of the non-obese[20]. When obese subjects are machine-fed with liquid diets, the daily calorie intake falls spontaneously to 25% or less of their normal daily requirements. Covert substitution of a liquid diet by fluids of reduced caloric density goes undetected and increases the energy deficit: when caloric dilution is achieved in obese patients by covertly replacing sucrose with aspartate in an otherwise normal diet, the energy intake falls by 25% without a compensatory increase in the volume of food ingested[21]. These preliminary findings suggest that a reduction in caloric density does not necessarily have an adverse effect on the palatability or acceptability of foodstuffs and for the future, may provide a useful means of reducing calorie intake.

Dietary fibre
It is difficult to overlook the possible relation between obesity and dietary fibre intake when obesity is so common in populations consuming a low-fibre diet and so rare in those taking a high-fibre diet[22]. Heaton (1973) has postulated that dietary fibre may serve as an obstacle to energy intake in several different ways[23]. Food fibre includes lignin, cellulose and hemi-cellulose, often termed unavailable carbohydrate. Volume for volume, fibre-rich foods provide less available energy than fibre-depleted foods. Their increased bulk and low calorie density may be advantageous in reducing energy intake by displacing foods of high calorie density from the diet. A man who replaced his average daily sucrose intake of 100 g iso-calorically with 2 lb of apples, might well find it very difficult to maintain his normal intake of other foods. Increased dietary fibre demands more chewing and has the effects of slowing food intake and reducing total intake by producing mild gastric distension and stimulating satiety. In addition, dietary fibre may reduce the efficiency of the small-bowel

absorptive processes by between 2 and 4%, and provides one possible explanation for the differences in carbohydrate and lipid metabolism observed in diets of differing fibre content[22]. At present, the role of a fibre-rich diet in the treatment of obesity is uncertain. The probable existence of a complex interrelationship between obesity, diabetes, coronary artery disease and dietary fibre intakes would suggest that attempts should be made to maintain an appropriate fibre intake whatever diet is chosen; in practice this is achieved cheaply and simply by the daily ingestion of small quantities of unprocessed bran.

Which dietary regimen?

Reducing diets which fulfil the criteria outlined above may be classified as inclusion or exclusion depending on whether or not a 'conventional' distribution of carbohydrate fat and protein content is maintained. Providing the total content does not fall below 800 kcal (3·3 MJ) per day, the intake of essential vitamins and nutrients is unlikely to be significantly less than recommended whichever regimen is chosen[24,25]. Weight reduction is directly related to daily energy deficit and there is no evidence that calories derived from carbohydrate, fat or protein differ in any significant way. Numerous metabolic studies suggest that the desirable minimum daily intake of protein is 15–25 g (provided this is of high biological value) and 30–45 g carbohydrate[26]. The adaptive responses necessary to conserve lean body mass reach their maximum efficiency after 2 weeks and result in equilibrium of nitrogen balance within 4 weeks. Providing the chosen regimen meets these requirements, significant ketosis and negative nitrogen balance will be avoided[26]. These minimum recommended intakes of protein and carbohydrate will usually be exceeded by a regimen which provides 800–1500 kcal (3·3–6·3 MJ) daily.

The low-carbohydrate diet

In its simplest form, this diet comprises the omission of one or two specific food items which from the dietetic history have been identified as inappropriate, and excessive calorie sources always of carbohydrate origin. Common examples include beer, soft drinks, chips, potato crisps and confectionery. In such cases, it is unnecessary to attempt a change of eating habit by any means other than omitting these foodstuffs from the diet (Table 2). For many, however, a more detailed change in eating pattern will be required and the regimen adopted is commonly referred to as a low-carbohydrate diet. This diet is synonymous with the free diet or modified Marriott diet and is comparable with the so-called high-fat diet and high-protein diet. From a survey of UK general practitioners, low-carbohydrate diets are the most often prescribed, their great advantage being simplicity, economy and the avoidance of having to weigh food[27].

Table 2 A simple low-carbohydrate exclusion diet*

CUT OUT COMPLETELY

Sugar, glucose, jam, marmalade, honey, syrup, sweets, chocolates, treacle, buns, cakes, sweet biscuits, chocolate biscuits, pastry, pies, tinned fruit, ice cream, lemonade, glucose drinks, beer, stout, wines, sherry.

TAKE AS DESIRED

Meat, fish, cheese, bacon, eggs, vegetables (except peas, beans and potatoes), clear soup, Oxo, Bovril, Marmite, tea and coffee (milk from allowance, no sugar), butter, margarine, cream.

TAKE IN MODERATION

Bread, rolls, scones, porridge, potatoes, plain biscuits, pudding cereals, breakfast cereals, soup, fruit, fruit juice.

Do not exceed 1 pint of milk daily

---

* This will provide an average daily carbohydrate intake of approximately 140 g and a total daily energy intake of 1500 kcal (6·3 MJ)

The principle of the regimen is that carbohydrate is restricted to 80–120 g daily without deliberate restriction of fat or protein intake. In practice, the diet does not result in any major increase in protein intake and often reduces fat intake[28]. The consumption of both pure and highly refined carbohydrates is severely restricted and the intake of moderate carbohydrate foodstuffs is controlled using the prescription of a number of carbohydrate exchanges in 10 g carbohydrate equivalents (Table 3). By comparison with an isocaloric diet high in carbohydrate, hunger is usually more completely abolished[29] and weight loss during the first 2 weeks is higher[30]. This reflects the changes in total body sodium and water following carbohydrate restriction[31]. However, after this initial period there is no significant difference between the rates of weight loss achieved by either regimen[32] and providing the carbohydrate content of the diet does not fall below a minimum of 30–45 g daily, neither regimen will induce hyperuricaemia[26]. Both diets have similar effects in lowering the plasma insulin and plasma lipids[31].

Total calorie restriction (inclusion diet)

A calorie-controlled or a mixed diet is the diet tried most often by men and women slimmers, and more than half consider it to be the best method for producing long-term weight loss[9]. Dietary advice regarding total calorie counting is based on the positive precepts of encouraging the consumption of most foods in moderation rather than the negative concept of banning certain foodstuffs. It may be particularly useful in subjects who fail to lose

Table 3 A 10 g carbohydrate exchange exclusion diet*

---

1 YOU MAY EAT AS MUCH AS YOU LIKE OF THESE

Meat, fish, bacon, ham, cheese, eggs
Vegetables, (except those mentioned below), lemon, rhubarb, fresh grapefruit
Clear soup, Oxo, Bovril, Marmite with vegetables added
Tea, coffee – milk from allowance but no sugar
Seasonings, herbs, spices
Butter, margarine, cream
Water, soda water, PLJ, tomato juice, diabetic or low-calorie squash

2 YOU MUST NOT EAT ANY OF THESE

Sugar, glucose, jam, marmalade, honey, syrup, treacle, sweets, chocolate
Buns, cakes, sweet biscuits, chocolate biscuits, pies, food coated in *batter* or *crumbs*
Tinned fruit in syrup, lemonade, glucose drinks, beer, stout, sweet wines, sweet sherry

3 YOU MAY HAVE . . . . . . OF THE FOLLOWING DAILY

½ slice bread – large loaf, white or brown
1 slice bread – small loaf, may be toasted
½ morning roll or small plain or wheaten scone
2 small tea biscuits, cream crackers, water biscuits, Cornish wafers, round oatcakes or crispbreads
1 digestive biscuit or large triangular oatcake
2 heaped tablespoons made porridge
3 tablespoons cornflakes, rice crispies or All-bran
1 Weetabix or Shredded Wheat
1 scoop or tablespoon potato, 1 medium-sized roast potato or 6 chips
2 tablespoons peas, baked or butter beans, parsnip or sweetcorn
Fruit: apple, pear, orange, fresh peach, small banana, 10–12 grapes, 2 large plums or 20 cherries
¾ cup of fruit juice – no added sugar
1 carton plain yoghurt or ½ carton fruit yoghurt
Small block or 1 scoop ice cream
3 tablespoons made-up jelly
Ladle thick soup, e g broth, lentil, tinned or packet soup
4 tablespoons milk pudding sweetened with Saxin
2 heaped teaspoons Ovaltine, Horlicks, cocoa
2 medium-sized sausages
3-inch square pastry

Allowance per day . . . . . . milk

4 OCCASIONALLY YOU MAY HAVE

Spirits, dry wine, dry sherry, light lager
Double cream

---

* 10 carbohydrate 'exchanges' and ½ pint of milk per day will provide approximately 120 g of carbohydrate and an energy intake of 1200 kcal (5 MJ)

weight on a low-carbohydrate diet, in persistent nibblers who rarely eat large meals, and in those who are unable to resist high-carbohydrate foods including alcohol. In practice, however, accurate calorie counting and recording are essential if success is to be achieved, and an almost obsessional approach in the weighing and measuring of food intake is required.

After the first 2 weeks of calorie restriction, the rate of weight loss achieved is similar to that of an isocaloric low-carbohydrate diet. On an 800 kcal (3·3 MJ) mixed diet, an increasing proportion of the energy deficit is derived from the body fat, the percentage rising from 93% to 98% within 4 weeks, and the total losses of protein and fat resulting from these two regimens are comparable[33].

'Formula' diets
'Formula' diets are radical alternatives to conventional diets. They comprise liquid food preparations which are intended to replace all other dietary intake. They include supplements of vitamins and minerals in addition to specified quantities of fat, carbohydrate and protein, and with strict compliance the patient's daily energy intake can be calculated very accurately. The successful use of one proprietary formula diet in patients with refractory obesity was reported by Seaton and Duncan (Metercal: Mead Johnson Ltd)[34]. A similar preparation of higher carbohydrate content (Carnation Slender: Carnation Foods Ltd) is currently available in Britain[35] and other products intended primarily to promote weight regain in cachetic states (e.g. Triosorbon) can be adapted for use in obesity. Few patients can tolerate a formula diet for more than a few weeks. There is no evidence to suggest that they will promote a permanent change in eating habit and therefore they are of little value in the long-term treatment of obesity. It seems possible that if they are of use, it is in the short-term 'control' of cosmetic obesity. A cheaper alternative is three pints of milk daily. The use of starvation and semi-starvation regimes is discussed elsewhere.

Results
Irrespective of the method of dieting, approximately half of the men and one-third of the women who completed the Consumers' Association questionnaire said that their chosen diet had become a permanent way of life, but this was particularly true of subjects taking an exclusion regimen. These were less distressed by hunger and lost more weight than dieters using the inclusion regimen, though the rate of weight loss tended to be slower[8]. Using such a carbohydrate-restricted diet the long-term results can be impressive, and Craddock has shown that one in four patients can achieve and maintain a loss of 10% of their initial weight for years[12]; a proportion similar to that observed in subjects attending a Slimming

Organisation[36]. Success is more frequent in men, in married individuals with children, in the less neurotic, in patients with a physical condition who will benefit by weight reduction and in those whose weight problem has been of less than 5 years duration[13].

However, the potential benefit from attempted weight control cannot be assessed purely in physical terms. An improvement in the quality of life may result from the identification and management of psychological problems, and in this respect every patient represents the unique problem of management.

OBESITY IN CHILDREN

General considerations

In children, as in adults, obesity has become a common nutritional disorder and may cause serious emotional and physical disabilities. The prevalence of childhood obesity is difficult to define but may be rising, particularly in the lower social classes, and may affect up to 9% of boys and 15% of girls. The assessment of weight changes in children is more difficult than in adults since these changes occur in the context of normal growth. Tanner *et al.* (1968) have shown that the normal growth rate doubles during puberty, and his standard tables are of considerable help in the assessment of the obese child[37]. Though obese children tend to be taller than the non-obese, their advanced bone age often ensures that their ultimate height is no greater than that of their peers and indeed, may be less[38].

The majority of obese children develop their obesity before the age of 6 years[39] and there seems little doubt that the obese child is more likely to become an obese adult than the non-obese child, particularly if the parents are obese[40]. One-third of obese adults develop their obesity at or before adolescence, confirming an important link between childhood and adult obesity[41].

The discovery that adults who became obese in childhood may have a greater fat-cell number than those whose obesity developed after adolescence encouraged the belief that obesity in adults might be preventable if fat-cell replication could be restricted by therapy during certain critical periods of development[42,43]. Serious doubt has now been cast on the validity of these observations, and the division of obesity into hypertrophic and hyperplastic types may be misleading[44,45]. Studies of the physical development in childhood in relation to the velocity of weight gain in infancy do not support the hypothesis that over-nutrition in infancy is a major determinant of subsequent obesity, and reveal that only 10% of overweight children can be identified prospectively[46].

In view of the increased incidence of respiratory disease, orthopaedic problems and psychiatric illness associated with paediatric and adolescent obesity, weight reduction in the obese juvenile is a desirable health goal[47]. The ideal dietary regimen should reduce weight steadily and maintain a weight reduction without incurring physical or psychiatric upset, reduction of lean body mass or impairment of normal growth velocity. Unfortunately, side-effects attributable to calorie restriction can occur, though their significance remains controversial. Stunkard and Mendelson claim that psychiatric problems may result from parental pressure on children to achieve weight loss[48]. Losses of lean body weight do occur during calorie restriction and are greater when dieting before puberty[49]. Subnormal growth rates have been recorded frequently in children undergoing weight reduction, the growth rate being moderately attenuated[50,51].

Dietary management of obese children

In general, the approach is little different from that employed in the management of the obese adult. The composition of the dietary regimen chosen is of secondary importance, providing that a daily energy deficit of 500 kcal (2·1 MJ) can be achieved with at least 15% of the calorie intake as protein and an adequate intake of essential nutrients. Though the evidence is inconclusive, trials using a high-protein/low-carbohydrate regimen appear to produce better results than a more conventional balanced diet[52].

The eating pattern of most young people in the Western World is such that many clinics confine their choice of diet to one of carbohydrate restriction and in this context an exchange-type regimen appeared to be the most suitable[53]. A low-carbohydrate diet using an exchange system will allow children to continue their snacking habits and may provide the framework for the development of a better and permanent eating habit. In addition, the preservation of a normal lifestyle using a low-carbohydrate diet should help reinforce the concept of normality and encourage persistence with weight reduction. In early childhood, the success of attempted calorie restriction will inevitably reflect the enthusiasm, co-operation and understanding of parents. By contrast, in early adolescence, additional difficulties are encountered and result from the normal rebellion against parental help and advice and the extreme dislike of appearing to be different in any way from their peer group. The adolescents' sensitivity with respect to weight, coupled with an increasing independence, may render them temporarily untreatable and, as such, the best that can be hoped for is that during this period of rapid growth, their weight will plateau. Fortunately, the going is much easier in mid- to late-teens; the difficulties imposed by obesity in realizing adult aspirations commonly result in a strong desire to lose weight, and make late adolescence the optimal period for attaining a desirable weight.

For the grossly obese child, conventional dietary advice has little to offer and in these distressed and distressing juveniles it is best to accept that if weight loss is to be obtained, a more radical approach will be required. A semi-starvation regimen using a protein-sparing technique will often secure most of the goals of the ideal weight-reducing regimen mentioned previously. Though some loss of lean tissue seems inevitable, no long-term deleterious effect on growth has yet been apparent and in the majority, significant weight losses can be achieved without hospital admission[47].

Results of dietary therapy

The published long-term results of dietary therapy are discouraging. There is no correlation between initial success and subsequent weight maintenance and only one in four children will achieve and maintain a weight reduction to within 20% of their desirable weight[54]. 60% of obese children in their early teens can be expected to remain obese 40 years later[55]. Even in late adolescence, the prognosis is not good[56] and it is possible that in future behavioural modifications, combined with a suitable dietary regimen, may improve the outlook for the obese child[57].

OBESITY IN PREGNANCY

General considerations

Two-thirds of obese women develop their obesity after their early teens, while only a minority become overweight after the age of 40[58]. This suggests that pregnancy and the rearing of children are important factors in the aetiology of obesity. For many, weight gain during pregnancy is excessive and not all the excess weight is lost after pregnancy; a cumulative effect can occur in the multiparous. In others, the change in lifestyle and social circumstances following a pregnancy results in a reduction in exercise and the boredom of being housebound may cause, or aggravate, a weight problem[8].

The antenatal supervision of a pregnancy is an opportune time to pursue preventive and therapeutic aspects of health care, including weight control. For most women the time is one of heightened awareness of health hazards, and the lessons learned could improve the dietary habits of both mother and family[59].

Normal weight gain in pregancy

Doctors accept that the pregnant woman should not be 'eating for two'. The extra energy requirement during the second and third trimesters of pregnancy amounts to only about 200 kcal (0.8 MJ) per day. The addition of half a pint of milk a day alone would provide the 36 000 kcal (151 MJ) necessary to sustain an entire pregnancy. It follows that intakes in excess of this modest requirement may rapidly lead to excessive weight gains during pregnancy.

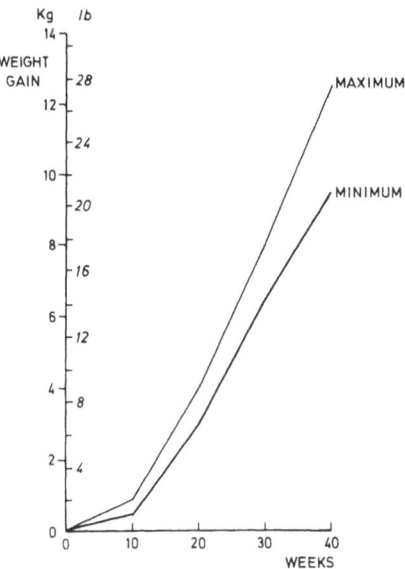

Figure 1 Weight gain during pregnancy for women of normal weight[8] (reproduced with the permission of the Consumers' Association)

The fetus, products of conception and maternal fluid changes in pregnancy contribute on average 3·4 kg (7½ lb), 2 kg (4½ lb), and 3·6 kg (8 lb) respectively during a normal pregnancy. A total loss of 9 kg (20 lb) can therefore be expected after delivery and in the early post-partum period[60]. Considerable differences of opinion surround the recommendation of a suitable total weight gain and the rate of weight gain during pregnancy (Figure 1). The figure gives a good idea of a suitable weight gain during the 40 weeks of pregnancy. The two lines show a reasonable minimum and maximum weight gain (this is not so much to account for the size in babies but rather reflects the somewhat different views among doctors). Since the average woman will gain between 10 and 12½ kg (22–28 lb) during pregnancy the resultant increase in body fat will be around 1–3·6 kg (2–8 lb). Given an average family size of two to three children if uncorrected, this increase in total body fat during the childbearing years could result in a woman's weight rising by up to 9 kg (20 lb). Thus maternal considerations concerning the recommended weight gain in pregnancy are of considerable importance if obesity is to be avoided during these years.

Obesity maternal risk factors
Pre-pregnancy obesity and excessive weight gain during pregnancy are both associated with an increased incidence of hypertension, pre-eclampsia and eclampsia[81]. The massively obese pregnant woman (bodyweight ≥ 114 kg (250 lb)) is disposed to an increased risk of mortality, diabetes

mellitus, pyelonephritis and dystocia compared with non-obese gravidae[62,63]. In addition, the sometimes irrational tendency to delay Caesarian section in the obese, when normally indicated, accounts in part for the increased maternal morbidity sometimes reported in association with obesity during delivery and in the puerperium[64].

Obesity: the fetal risk factors
Many studies have confirmed that big mothers have big babies. A comparison of maternal weight gain in pregnancy and fetal birth weight reveals a close correlation when total weight gains exceed 5 kg (11 lb)[65]. The pre-pregnancy weight is also directly associated with fetal birth weight, independent of weight gain during pregnancy[65]. Prematurity, i.e. a birth weight less than 2·5 kg (5½ lb), appears to be associated with an increased incidence of neonatal mortality and poor physical and mental development in the infant. Thus a low incidence of abnormal infant development is associated with high maternal weight gains during pregnancy, an effect which is apparently independent of other factors such as smoking or gestational age[66]. Since the birth weight is often a good prognostic index of neonatal well-being, it has been inferred by many that the heavier the mother before pregnancy, and the more weight she gains during pregnancy, the healthier her baby will be[67]. One extensive study of obese women during pregnancy concluded that maternal obesity was not associated with any significant increase in fetal morbidity or mortality[68]. However, women who are obese before pregnancy still tend to have larger, healthier babies even when they lose weight during pregnancy, and the highest incidence of prematurity occurs in infants whose mothers weigh less than 55 kg (120 lb) before pregnancy and gain less than 5 kg (11 lb) during pregnancy[65] (Table 4).

Aims in the management of obese and non-obese gravidae
The dietary advice given during pregnancy should recognize there is an apparent conflict of interest between maternal and fetal well-being. The review of nearly 12 000 pregnancies by Eastman and Jackson has provided a number of useful guidelines[65]. The independent influences of pre-pregnancy weight and weight gain during pregnancy on birth weight provide certain therapeutic advantages. There is no clinically significant difference in mean birth weights of infants from gravidae whose pregnancy weight was greater than 73 kg (160 lb) and who gained less than 5 kg (11 lb) during pregnancy and infants of non-obese gravidae who gained 10–12½ kg (22–28 lb)[65]. It follows that non-obese women should be encouraged to gain 10–12½ kg (22–28 lb) during pregnancy. The rate of weight gain should not exceed 1 lb per week during the second and third trimesters. However, when the pre-pregnancy weight indicates moderate obesity (20–29% in

Table 4 The relationship between pre-pregnancy weight, weight gain during pregnancy and fetal birth weight

Maternal group (Caucasians)	No.	Mean birth weight (g)	Cases with birth weight below 2501 g	
			No.	Percentage
High pre-pregnancy weight ⎫ High weight gain ⎭	58	3831	0	0·0
High pre-pregnancy weight ⎫ Low weight gain ⎭	132	3628	3	2·3
Low pre-pregnancy weight ⎫ High weight gain ⎭	328	3453	5	1·5
Low pre-pregnancy weight ⎫ Low weight gain ⎭	104	3044	6	5·8

Definitions: High pre-pregnancy weight = 72 kg (160 lb)
High weight gain = 14 kg (30 lb)
Low pre-pregnancy weight = 54 kg (120 lb)
Low weight gain = 5 kg (11 lb)

Date from Ref. 65, with permission of the Editors

excess of desirable weight), attempts should be made to restrict weight gain to between 5 and 9 kg (11–20 lb). When the pre-pregnancy weight is 30% or more in excess of desirable, weight gain can safely be restricted to less than 5 kg without any significant adverse changes in the incidence of prematurity. In the massively obese, the aim should be to prevent any weight gain.

Dietary management during pregnancy
Since the pre-pregnancy weight bears little relation to weight gain during pregnancy, every effort should be made to monitor, and when necessary correct, the rate of weight gain. Obese gravidae in the first trimester could be effectively reduced from the outset by using a simplified low-carbo-hydrate regimen designed to provide 1500 kcal daily and including 1 pint of milk per day (Table 2). In the second trimester, a weekly weight gain in excess of 1 lb (0·45 kg) reflects the accumulation of fat and indicates a need for dietary advice. In this context, a carbohydrate-restricted regimen providing 1500 kcal (6·3 MJ) daily again is usually effective. Sudden weight gain during the third trimester is due to the fluid retention of pre-eclampsia.

After delivery, breast-feeding should be encouraged since this may not only reduce the likelihood of neonatal ill health but the additional calorie requirements (400 kcal (1·7 MJ) per day) could assist weight reduction when indicated. Reducing regimens providing less than 60 g of protein daily and less than 1500 kcal (6·3 MJ) per day are not recommended in mothers who wish to breast-feed, because of the risk of the suppression of lactation.

The results of dietary therapy
The incidence of pre-eclampsia can be dramatically reduced by carbohydrate restriction in obese gravidae and in gravidae whose rate of weight gain is excessive in the second trimester[69]. In one series only 9% of gravidae gained more than $12\frac{1}{2}$ kg (28 lb) of whom half were found to have pre-eclampsia, and the majority of those patients with pre-pregnancy obesity achieved a significant net weight loss during pregnancy[59]. With care and regular supervision, obesity and excessive weight gains in pregnancy can be reduced without ill-effects either to mother or fetus and creates an opportunity for preventive medicine which should not be overlooked.

OBESITY AND DIABETES MELLITUS

Introduction
Obesity is overwhelmingly the most common disease found to co-exist with diabetes mellitus. The intimate relationship between the two conditions is poorly understood, but the association is exceedingly common and can be summarized as follows: 25% of obese subjects have significant impairment of glucose tolerance[70]; 80% of diabetics are aged over 45 when the disease becomes clinically apparent (maturity onset diabetes) and all but a few exhibit a more or less severe degree of obesity. They possess a pancreatic beta-cell mass which is functional but secretes inadequate insulin in relation to body weight. Insulin deficiency is relative rather than absolute and the equation of insulin secretion versus body weight can be made to balance if fat-cell mass can be reduced. Obesity in juvenile-onset diabetes is very much less common but co-exists in at least one fascinating variant; the so-called maturity-onset diabetes of young persons (MODY) describes the young, overweight diabetic who can be controlled without insulin, and in whom the condition has a clear-cut (autosomal dominant) mode of inheritance[71].

Dietary management is the most important and often the only treatment necessary for the obese diabetic. These patients should have every reason to be well-motivated. They suffer from a condition which is an unwelcome addition to obesity, is regarded as a 'respectable' illness to be taken seriously by the lay public and responds admirably to dietary measures. The symptoms of diabetes (thirst, polyuria, nocturia and especially pruritus) are a most unpleasant addition to the normal discomforts of the obese state. Carbohydrate intolerance in the obese diabetic may be abolished by substantial weight loss but may deteriorate further if weight loss is not achieved[72,73]. Virtually all obese diabetics have access to professional advice, from doctors and dietitians, in contrast to simple obesity where advice is predominantly from lay sources. Therefore there seem to be compelling reasons why a successful outcome of dietary treatments should be expected in maturity-onset diabetes.

The facts are very different and are only too well known. The adherence rate of obese diabetics to any kind of diet is frankly appalling. For example, in the National Health Survey conducted 10 years ago in the USA, 22% of diabetics claimed that they had never been given any dietary advice[74]. Another 25% had received a diet but said that they did not follow it, and just over half (53%) indicated that they were following a prescribed diet. The situation is no better in Britain, a recent urban survey finding that only 25% of diabetics consumed within 10% of the prescribed food intake, most exceeding it greatly, when their actual intakes were studied over a week[75]. The long-term effects of this kind of dietary neglect are ably summarized by the careful studies of the University Group Diabetes Programme[13] which demonstrated that 'dieting' for $4\frac{1}{2}$ years by a group of one thousand obese, maturity-onset diabetics resulted in a mean weight gain of around 1% and no improvement in diabetic control. If maturity-onset diabetes with obesity is ignored, a minority of elderly patients (probably around 10%) will eventually show signs of pancreatic-beta-cell exhaustion, will begin to lose weight involuntarily as hyperglycaemia and glycosuria become sustained and severe, and will ultimately need permanent treatment with exogenous insulin injections. In addition, there is increasing evidence to indicate that persisting and uncontrolled obesity enhances the risk of developing non-specific (macrovessel) diabetic complications[70], particularly in the presence of hyperlipoproteinaemia, which occurs in about half of all obese diabetics at the time of diagnosis[76].

It follows that the physician must make strenuous efforts to ensure that obese diabetics are aware of the importance of weight loss. Some physicians continue to take the cynical view that obese diabetics should be left to stew in their own juice, until uncontrolled symptoms and failure of endogenous insulin combine to cause weight loss and promote a proper frame of mind for serious dieting. Such attitudes seem at best to be inhumane and at worst frankly unethical.

Dietary management: general considerations

The three principles in the dietary management of the obese diabetic are to –

(i) reduce body weight and maintain it at the reduced level;
(ii) correct hyperglycaemia;
(iii) restore plasma lipoprotein levels to normal.

The best type of diet to achieve these objectives is controversial[77] and a variety of very different approaches is in use. In Europe and North America most emphasize the importance of restricting carbohydrate intake to around 40% of the total daily calories, while some are equally enthusiastic regarding restriction of dietary fat intake and the importance of increasing the ratio of dietary polyunsaturated : saturated fat with the aim of achieving normal serum cholesterol levels[78]. In contrast, clinicians in Eastern and tropical countries report excellent control of obese diabetics using diets with remarkably high carbohydrate content; 64% of daily caloric intake in one Japanese study[79] and more than 70% in diabetic clinics on the Indian sub-continent[80]. These conflicting approaches can be reconciled. All are agreed that the primary consideration is the restriction of total daily caloric intake in obese diabetics; the proportion of the intake provided by carbohydrate is of secondary importance. In certain ethnic groups, complex carbohydrate (e.g. rice) constitutes the majority of their diet – whether normal or a reducing regime. This is especially true of Third-world countries. If there is a shortage of proteins and fats, then carbohydrate is necessary to make up the daily caloric total. In other words, it would appear that obese diabetics are perfectly able to tolerate a high proportion of daily food intake as carbohydrate, provided that the total daily caloric intake is sufficiently reduced to promote weight loss. However, not only the quantity, but also the nature, of daily carbohydrate intake is important. The adverse effects of excessive consumption of highly refined, simple carbohydrates are self-evident[78]. Recent work indicates that different complex carbohydrates (that is, starches) elicit very different metabolic responses. For example, potatoes are as potent as dextrose in producing elevated postprandial glucose levels and eliciting high secretion of insulin; bread elicits lower responses; and rice provokes the lowest plasma glucose and insulin responses. Furthermore, these differences are accentuated in persons with impaired glucose tolerance[81]. These observations may explain the success of 'Asiatic'-type diets and seem sufficiently important to have immediate practical applications to current European practice. However, in affluent Western societies, excessive daily caloric intake almost invariably results from excessive consumption of refined carbohydrate, and the physician can advise vigorous restriction of starch in the knowledge that liberal supplies of fat and protein are available to his patient. In general terms, therefore, the approach to the obese diabetic will differ little from the treatment of the obese non-diabetic.

It is essential to obtain a proper dietary history from the patient. Many do not regard liquids as foodstuffs, and will not reveal the full extent of their carbohydrate consumption unless specifically asked. Thirst is a leading symptom of diabetes and is frequently quenched with drinks of high carbohydrate content: many obese diabetic women at the time of diagnosis are drinking 1 l or more of lemonade per day, each litre providing at least 100 g of carbohydrate. Diabetic men may prefer beer or lager, but unfortunately the lower carbohydrate content of these alcoholic beverages is more than compensated for by the quantity consumed. The daily carbohydrate intake in many obese diabetics is remarkable: a figure of 400–500 g is commonplace and urinary glucose loss may exceed 200 g daily despite the fact that the patient's weight is steady. An added difficulty for many obese diabetics results from the confusion regarding the wide range of foods and drinks which are sweetened with Sorbitol, fructose or Xylotol – the so-called diabetic sugars which are claimed to be 'safe' for diabetics. This claim is based mainly on the premise that significant hyperglycaemia does not occur after their ingestion, that their utilization is partly independent of insulin and that their absorption from the gut is slower than that of glucose, sucrose or maltose[82]. There is a natural but unfortunate tendency for obese diabetics to assume that these sugars are harmless substitutes for the 'dangerous' sugars they have been warned against and to consume them *ad libitum* without appreciating the extra calories they provide. Their use should be prohibited or severely restricted in patients requiring to lose weight. Similar considerations apply to the use of diabetic lager by heavy beer drinkers who wish to continue the habit; again it must be explained that alchohol is itself an excellent source of calories and that its consumption must be reduced if successful weight loss is to be achieved.

Dietary regimens
The three aims of dietary management in the obese diabetic can usually be fulfilled by one or other of two simple exclusion diets. The first is an unmeasured, unweighed, carbohydrate-restricted diet (Table 2). This diet is of most value in newly diagnosed diabetics who are moderately obese but less than 30% in excess of desirable weight, in those who have a single source of excess carbohydrate intake readily identified from the dietary history and in the elderly, especially with additional handicaps – such as failing vision and memory. This simple diet usually provides a daily carbohydrate intake of 130–150 g and a daily energy intake of about 1500 kcal (6·3 MJ). It should abolish the symptoms of hyperglycaemia and contain the modest degree of obesity exhibited by these patients.

The second diet has already been described (Table 3). It is a modified Marriott diet in which carbohydrate restriction is achieved by using 10 g exchanges which are specified in number but not distributed in a fixed pattern throughout the day. It is indicated for younger diabetics and for those who are greater than 30% in excess of desirable weight. In these obese diabetics, the daily calorie intake should be reduced sufficiently to achieve an energy deficit of at least 500–2000 kcal (2·1–4·2 MJ) per day, carbohydrate providing 40–50% of the calories. In practice, a safe principle is to prescribe 10 daily carbohydrate exchanges and limit the milk allowance to half a pint daily. It is important to emphasize to the patient that these exchanges can be distributed in any pattern throughout the day, and that their nature is entirely dependent upon individual preference. Experiments with carbohydrate foods which are not listed on the diabetic sheet should be initially discouraged. Frequent interviews with the dietitian or doctor may be necessary to resolve any difficulties, and a copy of the British Diabetic Association's guide[83] to the carbohydrate content of proprietary foods is invaluable for the persistent experimenter. After all, the guide was primarily intended for precisely such patients. A number of patients, particularly the elderly or the markedly overweight, are bewildered or uneasy with a flexible exchange type of diet. This usually becomes apparent during the first interview. These patients prefer a more rigid regimen which can be provided by a total calorie restricted (inclusion) diet of 1000–1200 kcal (4·2–5·0 MJ) per day.

The joint aims of treating obesity and diabetes by the same means should be clearly explained, and all patients, except for the blind, can be issued with a simple home test (Clinitest: Diastix: Testape) to monitor glycosuria and therefore success or failure in treating one aspect of their condition.

In assessing the response to dietary therapy, it is important to remember that correction of blood glucose, blood lipids and body weight abnormality do not occur simultaneously. The presence of diabetes will retard the initial velocity of weight loss. This is because at diagnosis, many diabetics are mildly sodium and water depleted as a result of polyuria. On reduction of the carbohydrate intake, the blood glucose will fall steeply towards normal within a week; urinary losses of glucose, sodium and water will consequently be dramatically reduced and the modest diuretic response seen in the obese non-diabetic after carbohydrate restriction will not been seen. In consequence, it is common to find that after 4 weeks of treatment, the body weight is unchanged and may even have increased though the blood glucose is almost normal and urine tests have remained negative for glucose. Prior explanation of this expectation may avoid the disillusionment of the patient and encourage persistance with the chosen dietary regimen. After 4 weeks of adherence to the diet, the rate of weight loss will be the same as that achieved in obese non-diabetics and no attempt should be made to reduce the calorie intake further until 8 weeks have elapsed and the situation has been carefully reassessed. Failure to appreciate these changes may lead the inexperienced clinician to misinterpret the lack of weight loss as dietary non-compliance; the patient will deny this with all the vigour of disappointment and honesty and the resulting mutual recriminations may destroy the doctor–patient rapport and discourage any further efforts to diet.

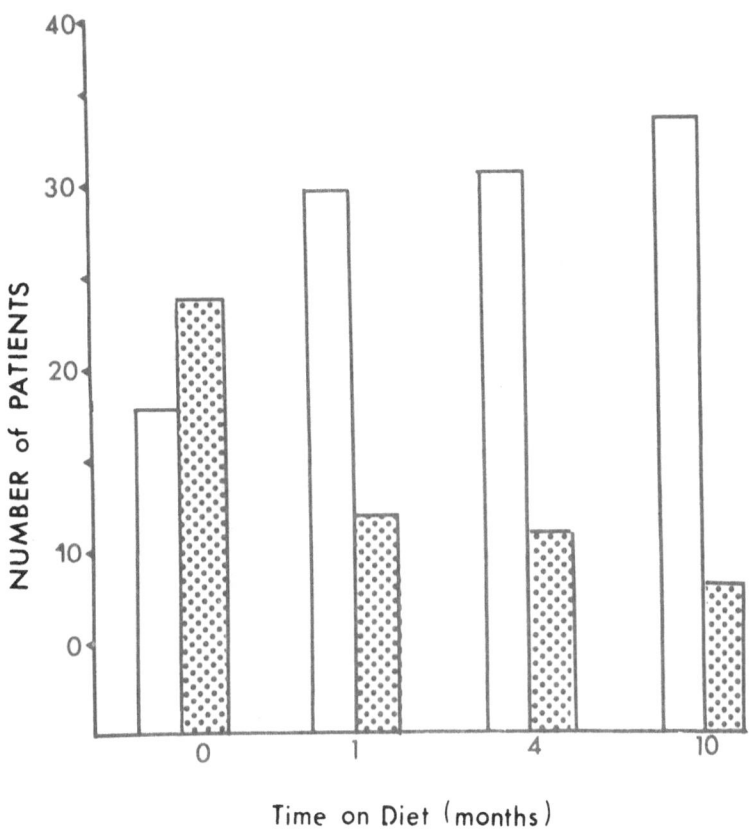

Figure 2 Effect of dietary carbohydrate restriction on lipoprotein abnormalities in obese patients with newly-diagnosed (maturity-onset) diabetes mellitus. Hyperlipoproteinaemia (shown by the shaded blocks) is common at time of diagnosis but lipoprotein levels fall within 1 month of dietary treatment and will usually remain normal as long as weight loss continues[76]. Open columns are normal values; hatched columns are elevated values.

The effects of dietary carbohydrate restriction on lipoprotein levels in a group of newly diagnosed obese diabetics treated by the exchange type of diet is shown in Figure 2. This illustrates the remarkable frequency of hyperlipoproteinaemias in these patients and demonstrates that both type II and type IV hyperlipoproteinaemias can be corrected without the use of drugs or complex diets designed to alter the amount and composition of dietary fat[76]. Once the blood lipid levels have returned to normal, they will only remain there if weight loss is maintained. The correction of hyperlipoproteinaemia may help check the excessive morbidity from degenerative vascular disease which is so common in obese diabetics. The knowledge that this can be achieved by simply restricting dietary carbo-hydrate should provide doctor and patient with a strong determination to succeed in promoting weight loss.

Results of treatment
Despite the benefits that may accrue from successful dieting, it is unfor-tunately true that the proportion of diabetics who succeed in losing sub-stantial quantities of weight is no different from that in non-diabetic obesity and some have suggested that it may even be less[84]. In many maturity onset diabetics the blood sugar returns to near normal but the obesity persists. However, efforts to promote weight loss by advising even more rigorous restriction of dietary carbohydrate or by changing to a calorie-controlled type of diet are usually unsuccessful. Drugs in the treatment of obesity are discussed elsewhere but the biguanide metformin is probably the only effective and safe oral hypoglycaemic agent that can be prescribed without expecting an increase in the patient's weight. The use of sulphonylurea drugs is almost invariably associated with some weight gain and this may limit their value in obese diabetics. There are other factors which determine the choice of an oral hypoglycaemic agent; the risk of enhancing or perpetuating obesity may take second place to the need to relieve distressing symptoms such as polyuria and pruritus, especially in the elderly, or to conserve residual beta-cell function in patients with marked hyperglycaemia. Fenfluramine has been suggested as a particularly suitable anorexic drug for these patients[85] but its direct effect on blood glucose level is so small that it cannot be seriously regarded as an oral hypoglycaemic and its use in uncontrolled diabetes is primarily as an anti-obesity agent. Another interesting approach has been to accept that many patients find it impossible to make the necessary reduction in carbohydrate intake and instead to limit the absorption of carbohydrate by incorporating into the diet a quantity of dietary fibre in palatable form such as guar. This reduces glycosuria in diabetics[86] but in practice, it has proved extremely difficult for patients to find foodstuffs containing quan-tities of guar: the treatment is still at the stage of clinical trials but may have more widespread application if food manufacturers ever market a range of guar-containing products on a large scale.

In summary, the dietary treatment of the obese diabetic is generally disappointing as regards weight loss but usually satisfactory in lowering blood sugar and relieving the symptoms of uncontrolled diabetes. Unfor-tunately, it does not appear that reduction of hyperglycaemia alone protects these patients in any degree from the development of vascular disease, and persisting obesity will be accompanied by significant hyperlipopro-teinaemia in a high percentage of patients. A satisfactory treatment for the overweight diabetic is a major clinical problem. Continuing efforts to promote weight loss should not be readily abandoned. The dietary manage-ment of the obese diabetic remains a compromise between the patient's expressed desires and the profession's aim to control the diabetic condition with all its associated risk factors.

OBESITY AND THE HEART

Introduction
Obesity is an important contributory factor in cardiovascular morbidity and mortality. The increased risk is largely mediated by the accom-panying pathological traits which include impared glucose tolerance, hypertension and hyperlipoproteinaemia. In addition, obesity may have a unique and independent effect in angina pectoris in men and in cardiac failure and cerebral infarction in women[93]. Though it is difficult to estimate the precise net and joint importance of obesity and its associated risk factors in relation to cardiovascular disease, it seems reasonable to assume that since weight reduction reduces these risk factors, dietary manipulation and weight control will result in a general improvement in cardiovascular health. Judging by the effects of weight loss on atherogenic traits, a 20% reduction in the weight of young obese individuals could result in a 40% reduction in the risk of coronary heart disease (CHD) and might improve considerably the exercise tolerance and quality of life in patients with angina pectoris or cardiac failure[87].

The role of dietary factors in coronary heart disease

Dietary fat
The evidence linking dietary fat to the incidence of CHD reveals that major significant correlations are to be found in association with the dietary intake of saturated fatty acids and triglycerides rather than dietary cholesterol or total dietary fat[88]. Diets high in saturated fat are usually high in cholesterol and the average daily diet will contain roughly 1·3 mmol (500 mg) of cholesterol. At this level of consumption, 60% of dietary cholesterol is absorbed, though with higher intakes the absorption rate falls to about 30%. Genetic influences are considered to be the major controlling factors in this process; a grossly elevated cholesterol intake is required before any change in plasma cholesterol concentration occurs and even then only a transient effect is observed[89].

The deposition of cholesterol within the arterial wall is influenced by the concentrations of cholesterol-rich low-density lipoproteins (LDL) and high density lipoproteins (HDL). HDL appears to prevent excess cholesterol deposition and its plasma concentration correlates negatively with the incidence and mortality of CHD[90,91]. The fatty acid composition of adipose tissue is known to reflect long-term dietary habits. The percentage of linoleic acid (an essential polyunsaturated fatty acid) in plasma and adipose tissue has been shown to be particularly low in patients with CHD[92]. It has also been suggested that diets with low polyunsaturated : saturated fat (P : S) ratios may increase the incidence of CHD and are associated with reduced plasma concentrations of HDL[93].

Dietary carbohydrate
The different insulin responses to a variety of carbohydrates have been discussed in the management of the obese diabetic and illustrate the possible advantages and disadvantages of certain carbohydrate foodstuffs in the control of glucose tolerance and plasma lipids[81]. Studies of HDL metabolism in man have shown that diets high in carbohydrate may increase HDL catabolism without change in synthesis rate, suggesting that high-carbohydrate diets might confer an increase atherogenic risk[94]. Epidemiological studies have implicated dietary sucrose as an aetiological factor in atherogenesis[95]. However, many disagree, and in studies of patients with CHD and controls no difference has been found in sucrose intakes[96], but dietary fat and sucrose intakes may be closely related and when corrections are made for this, the initial correlation between sucrose intakes and CHD mortality is lost[97]. It seems likely that the dietary saturated fat intake is a more important contributor, though dietary sucrose may have significant additive effect. Sucrose has been shown to be a potent inducer of the enzymes fatty acid synthetase and saturase, while linoleic acid, an essential fatty acid, is known to be a major repressor of these enzymes. Thus, it is conceivable that diets rich in sucrose and deficient in polyunsaturated fats (and therefore linoleic acid) may prove to be particularly atherogenic, though this is still unproven in man[93].

Dietary fibre
Epidemiological studies suggest that CHD may be associated with low intakes of dietary fibre[98]. No clear underlying mechanism has been isolated to account for this association, and while different dietary fibres have been shown in animals to have different effects on the plasma lipids, studies in man have been equivocal[99]. More recently, men who consume a higher dietary fibre intake from cereals rather than from fruit and vegetables, have been shown to have a lower incidence of CHD[98]. In the same study, the incidence of CHD in men appeared inversely related to calorie intake, a finding which may reflect differences in physical activity and energy expenditure as well as differences in dietary cereal fibre intake.

It has been suggested that cereal fibre, being rich in polyunsaturated fat, may be the vehicle for essential nutrients like linoleic acid, and the low fibre content of modern, westernized diet could be one of the many factors contributing to the present epidemic of CHD[98].

Summary
Primary prevention trials suggest that reducing dietary saturated fat and substituting polyunsaturated fats may reduce the incidence of CHD[8]. It remains to be shown whether the correction of the lipid disturbances seen frequently in patients with CHD will eventually affect the incidence of CHD among the younger population. Most agree that weight reduction is of primary importance in the obese patient with CHD, and the exact constituents of the diet are of relatively minor importance. Similarly, weight reduction, and stopping smoking, should be the initial steps in the management of the obese patient with diabetes, hypertension or hyperlipo-proteinaemia. At present, the evidence is insufficient to warrant a change in the normal dietary constituents of the whole community. However, until proof of efficacy is available, it would seem prudent to take adequate dietary fibre and to avoid high sucrose and high saturated fat intakes, particularly in the young non-obese patient with a family history of CHD, hyperlipoproteinaemia or multiple risk factors[100,101].

OBESITY AND HYPERLIPOPROTEINAEMIA

General considerations
Hyperlipoproteinaemia (HLP) is a major consequence of obesity, and may account in part for the excess cardiovascular risk of obese individuals. In a study of men aged less than 50 with angiographically proven coronary artery disease, obesity and hypertriglyceridaemia were found in 71% and 49% respectively and appeared the commonest risk factors associated with CHD[105]. Though HLP is not an invariable outcome of obesity, the reported incidence of HLP in the obese is high, as is the incidence of obesity in patients with HLP, particularly type IV[106]. While obesity has only been shown to have a marginal effect of the plasma cholesterol concentration, the degree of adiposity appears to be directly related to the total body cholesterol stores and turnover rate[107]. The increase in lipolysis resulting from increased body fat, and the altered regulation of lipolysis in the obese, accounts for the recognized relationship between degree of adiposity and plasma triglyceride concentration. The excess plasma lipid of obese individuals is transported predominantly in the very low-density lipoprotein (VLDL) fraction, which may be associated with a reduced cholesterol content in other lipoproteins, notably HDL[107].

Treatment

Until evidence to the contrary is available, HLP, whether primary or secondary, will require treatment in the young patient with or without obesity, and in all instances the diet remains the keystone of effective therapy – see Table 5[108] and Table 6[109]. Although the optimal dietary composition is controversial, most are agreed that when HLP and obesity co-exist, the primary aim in therapy is directed towards weight reduction. Hypertriglyceridaemia (types IIB, III, IV and V) will respond readily to weight reduction in the obese and often is most effectively secured using a low-carbohydrate regimen. Caloric restriction is considerably less effective in hypercholesterolaemia and in types I and IIA HLP a low-fat diet will be required.

Table 5　The classification of the hyperlipoproteinaemias

Type	Lipid abnormality	Lipoprotein abnormality	Lipid group	Obesity	Glucose tolerance
I	Cholesterol E	Chylomicrons (+++)	D	Occasional	Occasional
IIA	Cholesterol E Triglyceride N	LDL↑ (B–LP)	B	Occasional	Occasional
IIB	Cholesterol E Triglyceride E	LDL↑ VLDL↑ (pre B–LP)	D	Common	Common
III	Cholesterol E Triglyceride E	B–VLDL↑ (Broad B–LP)	D	Very Common	Very Common
IV	Cholesterol N(E) Triglyceride E	VLDL↑	C, D	Very Common	Very Common
V	Cholesterol E Triglyceride E	Chylomicrons (+) VLDL↑	D	Very Common	Very Common

N=normal; E=elevated; LDL=low-density lipoprotein; VLDL=very low-density lipoproteins; B–LP = beta-lipoproteins
Data from Ref. 108, with permission of the Editors

Though proof of efficacy is still lacking, effective dietary treatment may retard the premature development of atherosclerosis and will usually relieve the uncommon complications of hypertriglyceridaemia, mainly xanthomas and abdominal pain in types I and V HLP. In most instances, the use of the diets outlined in Table 6 will reduce the plasma triglyceride concentration by as much as 60%, and the plasma cholesterol by up to

Table 6 Dietary regimens in the management of the hyperlipoproteinaemias

Dietary Factor	Type I	Type IIA	Type IIB	Type III	Type IV	Type V
Calories	Normal	Normal	Restricted in obesity	Restricted in obesity	Restricted in obesity	Restricted in obesity
Carbohydrate	Normal	Normal	Control (no sucrose) 40%–50% of	Control (no sucrose) calorie intake	Control (no sucrose) as carbohydrate	Control (no sucrose)
Fat	All fat restricted to 35 g daily	Control intake of saturated fat		Restrict to 40% of calories and control intake of saturated fat	Control intake of saturated fat	Restrict to 30% of calories and restrict intake of saturated fat
Cholesterol rich food (Eggs and dairy produce)	Normal	As little as possible (meat only)			Moderate restriction	
Alcohol	Avoid completely	Normal	Limited	Limited	Limited	Avoid completely

Data from Ref. 109, with permission of the Author and Editors

30%, within a month in in-patients with type IV HLP. However, in asymptomatic out-patients compliance is often poor, and the results of dietary therapy are much more disappointing[110].

OBESITY AND HYPERTENSION

General considerations

The evidence relating the incidence of hypertension to obesity is impressive, and it has been estimated that control of obesity might reduce the prevalence of hypertension by 50%[102]. Dahl (1972) suggested that the reduction in blood pressure following weight loss was the result of salt, rather than calorie, restriction and claimed that significant reductions in blood pressure occurred only after weight had fallen to below desirable weight[103]. However, it has now been shown that successful weight reduction in obese hypertensives will result in a substantial improvement in blood pressure control independent of dietary sodium intake[11,104]. In the first of these studies, hypertensive patients whose body weight was on average 30% in excess of desirable were reviewed; of these 81 received dietary advice designed to reduce the daily calorie intake to 800–1000 kcal (3·4–4·2 MJ) without conscious salt restriction. All patients lost at least 3 kg (7 lb) in weight over a 4-month period, and all but two achieved a clinically significant reduction in blood pressure[11]. The mean initial weight of these patients was 85 kg (187 lb) and a mean weight loss of approximately 10 kg (22 lb) was achieved, resulting in a 20% reduction in mean systolic and diastolic pressures; on average, the blood pressure fell from 168/111 mmHg to 134/89 mmHg. No changes in treatment were necessary in those patients already taking hypotensive drugs, and the changes in weight and blood pressure were all highly significant when compared with a control group of obese hypertensives who were not given dietary advice.

In the second of these studies, 67 obese hypertensive patients were included in the trial, and of these 49 were available for analysis 1 year later. The initial mean percentage excess weight was 6% and mean blood pressure 167/102 mmHg. Dietary advice was randomly allocated and comprised one of three schedules; an 800 kcal (3.4 MJ) balanced diet and referral to a dietitian, an 800 kcal (3.4 MJ) diet sheet with simple instructions by the physician or just simple encouragement to lose weight with appropriate advice without the use of either diet sheet or the dietetic services. The mean weight losses achieved over the year were 5 kg (11 lb), $2\frac{1}{2}$ kg (5·5 lb) and 2 kg (4·5 lb) respectively. One-third had lost 6 kg (13 lb) or more, required fewer increases in hypotensive drug therapy and achieved a considerable improvement in blood pressure control. The net mean fall in blood pressure was 23/15 mmHg in those patients who lost weight compared with those who did not when drug therapy remained unchanged[104]. Providing the dietary programme is tailored to meet the patient's needs and lifestyle, compliance does not appear to be a major problem in planned weight reduction[11,101]. Weight control offers an efficient, cost-effective means of achieving blood pressure control in these patients, and may confer additional advantages by improving glucose tolerance and controlling the plasma lipids. By reducing the requirement for hypotensive drugs, and this minimizing side-effects, weight control should be the initial step in the management of obese hypertensives and can be expected to produce a reduction in blood pressure in the order of 3/2 mmHg per kg of weight lost.

SUMMARY OF THE DIETARY MANAGEMENT OF OBESITY AND ITS ASSOCIATED HEALTH PROBLEMS

Dietary advice is one vital aspect of the management of obesity and its associated problems, but its influence extends far beyond its effect on body weight. When assessed by weight loss alone, the success rate achieved by dietary management is disappointing. However, the additional potential benefits can be considerable. If success is defined as an improvement of all or some of the physical and psychological factors attendant upon obesity, then it can only be regularly achieved by those who combine a genuine interest in the problems of the obese with a sympathetic approach and are prepared to offer prolonged support and advice.

Each obese subject poses a unique problem of management and in some, obesity is no more than symptomatic of underlying distress. In others, it may be more appropriate to direct attention to a co-existent health hazard, e.g. smoking, before recommending weight reduction. If weight loss is advised, the first essentials are to establish a satisfactory rapport with the patient, assess motivation and reinforce realistic concepts of the anticipated rate of weight loss. A simple dietary regimen should be selected; one which is compatible with the patient's lifestyle and may effect a permanent change in energy balance. Attempts to assist the patient in weight reduction should not be abandoned readily, but it may ultimately be more advisable to encourage the patients to accept their obese state than to badger them against their better judgment to try again.

References

1 Osancova, K. and Hejda, S. (1975). Epidemiology of obesity. In T. Silverstone (ed.). *Obesity: Its Pathogenesis and Management*, p. 57. (Lancaster: MTP Press).

2 Ashwell, M. A. (1973). A survey investigating patients' view on doctors' treatment of obesity. *Practitioner*, **211**, 653

3 Ford, M. J., Scorgie, R. E. and Munro, J. F. (1977). Anticipated rate of weight loss during dieting. *Int. J. Obesity*, **1**, 239

4 Munro, J. F. (1973). The management of obesity. *Br. J. Hosp. Med.*, **10**, 8

5 Atkinson, R. L., Greenway, F. L., Bray, G. A., Dahms, W. T., Molitch, M. E., Hamilton, K. and Rodin, J. (1977). Treatment of obesity: comparison of physician and non-physician therapists using placebo and anorectic drugs in a double-blind trial. *Int. J. Obesity*, **1**, 113

6 Stuart, R. B. and Goire, K. (1978). Some correlates of the maintenance of weight loss through behaviour modification. *Int. J. Obesity*, **2**, 225

7 Innes, J. A., Campbell, I. W., Campbell, C. J., Needle, A. L. and Munro, J. F. (1974). Long term follow up of therapeutic starvation. *Br. Med. J.*, **2**, 356

8 Rudingo, E. (ed.). (1978). *Which? Way to Slim.* (London: Consumers Assoc.)

9 Rodin, J., Bray, G. A., Atkinson, R. L., Dahms, W. T., Greenway, F. L., Hamilton, K. and Molitch, M. (1978). Predictors of successful weight loss in an out-patient obesity clinic. *Int. J. Obesity*, **1**, 79

10 Silverstone, J. T. and Solomon, T. (1965). Psychiatric and somatic factors in the treatment of obesity. *J. Psychosom. Res.*, **9**, 249

11 Reisin, E. Abel, R., Modan, M., Silverberg, D. S., Eliahou, H. and Modan, B. (1978). Effect of weight loss without salt restriction on the reduction of blood pressure in overweight hypertensive patients. *N. Engl. J. Med.*, **298**, 1

12 Craddock, D. (1977). The free diet: 150 cases personally followed up after 10–18 years. *Int. J. Obesity*, **1,** 127

13 Goldner, M. G., Knatterud, G. L. and Prout, T. E. (1971). Effects of hypoglycaemic agents on vascular complications in patients with adult-onset diabetes. *J. Amer. Med. Assoc.*, **218,** 1400

14 Berchtold, P., Berger, M., Greiser, E., Dohse, M., Irmscher, K., Gries, F. A. and Zimmerman, H. (1977). Cardiovascular risk factors in gross obesity. *Int. J. Obesity*, **1,** 219

15 Dept. of Health and Social Security (1969). *Reports on Public Health and Medical Subjects*, No. 120. (London: HMSO)

16 Gordon, E. A. (1975). Treatment of obesity in the community – a consultative service. In A. Howard (ed.). *Recent Advances in Obesity Research*, vol. 1, p. 307. (London: Newman)

17 Fabry, P., Fodor, J., Heje, Z., Braun, T. and Zvolankova, K. (1964). The frequency of meals: its relation to overweight hypercholesterolaemia and decreased glucose tolerance. *Lancet*, **ii,** 614

18 Seaton, D. A. and Duncan, L. J. P. (1964). Treatment of 'refractory obesity' with a diet of two meals a day. *Lancet*, **ii,** 612

19 Munro, J. F., Seaton, D. A. and Duncan, L. J. P. (1966). Treatment of 'refractory obesity' with a diet of five meals a day. *Br. Med. J.*, **1,** 950

20 Van Itallie, T. B. (1978). Diets for weight reduction: mechanisms of action and physiological effects. *Int. J. Obesity*, **2,** 113

21 Porikos, K. P., Booth, G. and Van Itallie, T. B. (1977). Effect of covert nutritive dilution on the spontaneous food intake of obese individuals: a pilot study. *Am. J. Clin. Nutr.*, **30,** 1638

22 Trowell, H. (1975). Obesity in the western world. *Plant Foods for Man*, **1,** 157

23 Heaton, K. W. (1973). Food fibre as an obstacle to energy intake. *Lancet*, **ii,** 1418

24 Stock, M. and Yudkin, J. (1970). Nutrient intake of subjects on low carbohydrate diet used in the treatment of obesity. *Am. J. Clin. Nutr.*, **23,** 948

25 Amos, A. J. (1975). Cereals and obesity. In A. Howard (ed.). *Recent Advances in Obesity Research*, vol. 1, p. 296. (London: Newman).

26 Baird, I. McLean, Parsons, R. L. and Howard, A. N. (1974). Clinical and metabolic studies of chemically defined diets in the management of obesity. *Metabolism*, **23,** 645

27 Yudkin, J. (1968). Doctors' treatment of obesity: analysis of *The Practitioner* questionnaire. *Practitioner*, **201,** 330

28 Yudkin, J. (1974). The low-carbohydrate diet. In W. L. Burland, P. D. Samuel and J. Yudkin (eds.). *Obesity*, p. 271. (London: Churchill Livingstone)

29 Yudkin, J. and Carey, M. (1960). The treatment of obesity by the 'high fat' diet: the inevitability of calories. *Lancet*, **ii,** 939

30 Kekwick, A. and Pawan, G. L. S. (1956). Calorie intake in relation to body weight changes in the obese. *Lancet*, **ii,** 155

31 Lewis, S. B., Wallin, J. D., Kane, J. P. and Gerich, J. E. (1977). Effect of diet composition on metabolic adaptations to hypocaloric nutrition: comparison of high carbohydrate and high fat isocalorie diets. *Am. J. Clin. Nutr.*, **30,** 160

32 Pilkington, T. R. E., Gainsborough, H., Rosevoer, V. M. and Carey, M. (1960). Diet and weight reduction in the obese. *Lancet*, **i,** 856

33 Van Itallie, T. B., Yang, M. and Hashim, S. A. (1975). Dietary approaches to obesity: metabolic and appetitive considerations. In A. Howard (ed.). *Recent Advances in Obesity Research*, vol. 1, p. 256. (London: Newman), 256

34 Seaton, D. A. and Duncan, L. J. P. (1963). Treatment of 'refractory obesity' with 'formula' diet. *Br. Med. J.*, **2,** 219

35 Millar, J. W., Innes, J. A. and Munro, J. F. (1978). An evaluation of the efficacy and acceptability of 'Slender' in refractory obesity. *Int. J. Obesity*, **2,** 53

36 Garrow, J. S. (1975). A survey of three slimming and weight control organisations in the U.K. In A. Howard (ed.). *Recent Advances in Obesity Research*, vol. 1, p. 301. (London: Newman)

37 Tanner, J. M., Whitehouse, R. H. and Takaishi, M. (1966). Standards from birth to maturity for height, weight, height velocity and growth velocity; British children, 1965. *Arch. Dis. Childh.*, **41,** 454

38 Brook, C. G. D. (1973). Fat children. *Br. J. Hosp. Med.*, **10,** 30

39 Asher, P. (1966). Fat babies and fat children. The prognosis of obesity in the very young. *Arch. Dis. Childh.*, **41,** 672

40 Mayer, J. (1966). Some aspects of the problem of regulation of food intake and obesity. *N. Engl. J. Med.*, **274,** 610, 662

41 Mullins, A. G. (1958). The prognosis of juvenile obesity. *Arch. Dis. Childh.*, **33,** 307

42 Brook, C. G. D. (1974). Critical periods of childhood obesity. In W. L. Burland, P. Samuel and J. Yudkin, (eds.). *Obesity*, p. 85. (London: Churchill Livingstone)

43 Hager, A., Sjostrom, L., Arvidsson, B., Bjorntorp, P. and Smith, U. (1978). Adipose tissue cellularity in obese schoolgirls before and after dietary treatment. *Am. J. Clin. Nutr.*, **31,** 68

44 Hirsch, J. and Batchelor, B. (1976). Adipose tissue cellularity in human obesity. In M. J. Albrink (ed.). *Clinics in Endocrinology and Metabolism – Obesity*, vol. 5, p. 299. (Philadelphia: Saunders)

45 Jung, R. T., Gutt, M. I., Robinson, M. P. and James, W. P. (1978). Does adipocyte hypercellularity in obesity exist ? *Br. Med. J.*, **2,** 319

46 Mellbin, T. and Vuille, J. C. (1973). Physical development at 7 years of age in relation to velocity of weight gain in infancy with special reference to the incidence of overweight. *Br. J. Prev. Soc. Med.*, **27,** 225

47 Merritt, R. J. (1978). Treatment of pediatric and adolescent obesity. *Int. J. Obesity*, **2,** 207

48 Stunkard, A. and Mendelson, M. (1967). Obesity and the body image: 1. Characteristics of disturbances in the body image of some obese persons. *Am. J. Psychiat.*, **123,** 1296

49 Heald, F. P. and Hunt, S. M. (1963). Caloric dependence in obese adolescents as affected by degree of maturation. *J. Pediatr.*, **66,** 1035

50 Wolff, O. H. (1955). Obesity in childhood. *Q. J. Med.*, **24,** 109

51 Brook, C. G. D., Lloyd, J. K. and Wolff, O. H. (1974). Rapid weight loss in children. *Br. Med. J.*, **2,** 44

52 Howard, A. N., Dub, I. and McMahon, M. (1971). The incidence, cause and treatment of obesity in Leicester school children. *Practitioner*, **207,** 662

53 Meyer, E. E. and Newmann, C. G. (1977). Management of the obese adolescent. *Ped. Clin. N. Amer.*, **24,** 123

54 Lloyd, J. K., Wolff, O. H. and Whelan, W. S. (1961). Childhood obesity and long term study of height and weight. *Br. Med. J.*, **2,** 145

55 Abraham, S., Collins, G. and Nordsieck, M. (1971). Relationship of childhood weight status to morbidity in adults. *Publ. Health Reports*, **86,** 273

56 Stunkard, A. and Burt, A. (1967). Obesity and the body image: II. Age at onset of disturbance in the body image. *Am. J. Psychiat.*, **123,** 1443

57 Jordan, H. and Levitz, L. (1975). Behavior modification in the treatment of obesity. In W. Wimick (ed.). *Childhood Obesity*, (New York: Wiley)

58 Christakis, G. (1967). Community programs for weight reduction: experience of the Bureau of Nutrition, New York City. *Can. J. Publ. Health*, **58,** 499

59 Craddock, D. (1977). *Obesity and its Management*, 3rd edn. (London: Churchill Livingstone)

60 Hytten, F. E. and Leitch, J. (1969). *The Physiology of Human Pregnancy*, 2nd edn. (Oxford: Blackwell).

61 Peckham, C. H. and Bristianson, R. E. (1971). The relationship between pre-pregnancy weight and certain obstetric factors. *Am. J. Obstet. Gynecol.*, **111,** 1

62 Tracey, T. A. and Miller, G. L. (1969). Obstetric problems of the massively obese. *Obstet. Gynecol.*, **33,** 204

63 Maeder, E. C., Barno, A. and Mecklenburg, F. (1975). Obesity: a maternal high-risk factor. *Obstet. Gynecol.*, **45,** 669

64 Sicuranza, B. J. and Tisdall, L. H. (1975). Caesarian section in the massively obese. *J. Reprod. Med.*, **14,** 10

65 Eastman, N. J. and Jackson, E. (1968). Weight relationships in pregnancy. *Obstet. Gynecol. Survey*, **23,** 1003

66 Singer, J. E., Westphail, M. and Niswander, K. (1968). Relationships of weight gain during pregnancy to birth weight and infant growth and development in the first year of life. *Obstet. Gynecol.*, **31,** 417

67 Travers, C. K. (1976). Obesity and Pregnancy: A review. *Obesity and Bariatric Med.*, **5,** 172

68 Witten, S. B. (1958). Labor in the obese patient. *Obstet. Gynecol.*, **12,** 99

69 Hamlin, R. H. J. (1952). The prevention of eclampsia and pre-eclampsia. *Lancet*, **1,** 64

70 Keen, H. (1975). The incomplete story of obesity and diabetes mellitus. In A. Howard (ed.). *Recent Advances in Obesity Research*, vol. 1, p. 116. (London: Newman)

71 Tattershall, R. B. and Fajans, S. S. (1975). A difference between the inheritance of classical juvenile-onset and maturity-onset diabetes of young people. *Diabetes*, **24**(1), 44

72 Berger, M., Baumhoff, E. and Gries, F. A. (1975). Effect of weight reduction upon glucose tolerance in obesity. A follow up study of five years. In A. Howard (ed.). *Recent Advances in Obesity Research*, vol. 1, p. 128. (London: Newman)

73 Kataoka, K., Kvo, M., Nakajima, M., Yasuda, M. and Matsuki, S. (1975). Obese diabetics and their treatment. In A. Howard (ed.). *Recent Advances in Obesity Research*, vol. 1, p. 140. (London: Newman)

74 Holland, W. M. (1968). The diabetes supplement of the *National Health Service Journal of the American Dietetic Assoc.*, **52,** 387

75 Tunbridge, R. and Wetherill, J. H. (1970). Reliability and costs of diabetic diets. *Br. Med. J.*, **2,** 78

76 Thomson, J. E., Ballantyne, F., Scobie, I. N., Manderson, W. G. and MacCuish, A. C. (1978). Effect of dietary carbohydrate restriction on lipoprotein abnormalities in maturity onset diabetes mellitus. British Diabetic Assoc. (Medical and Scientific Section) Spring meeting

77 Editorial (1974). Diet for diabetics. *Lancet*, **i,** 398

78 Bierman, E. L., Albrink, M. J., Arky, R. A., Connor, W. T., Dayton, S., Spritz, N. and Steinberg, D. (1971). Principles of nutrition and dietary recommendation for patients with diabetes mellitus. *Diabetes*, **20,** 633

79 Bush, O. B. and Moriwaki, T. (1966). Diet and diabetes mellitus. In J. C. Patel and N. G. Talwalker (ed.). *Diabetes in the Tropics*, p. 533

80 Patel, J. C., Metha, A. B. and Dhirawani, M. K. (1969). High carbohydrate diet in the treatment of diabetes mellitus. *Diabetologia*, **5,** 243

81 Crapo, P. A., Reaven, G. and Olefsky, J. (1977). Postprandial plasma glucose and insulin response to different complex carbohydrates. *Diabetes*, **26,** 1178

82 Menhert, H. and Forster, H. (1965). Speed of absorption of different sugars and polyols in rats and normal probands. *Gastroenterologia*, **104** (suppl.), 101

83 British Diabetic Association (1977). Carbohydrate countdown. (Editorial) 1970. The overweight child. *Br. Med. J.*, **1,** 64

84 Balzola, F. and Palmo, A. (1975). The influence of metabolic disorders on weight loss of an obese caseload. In A. Howard (ed.). *Recent Advances in Obesity Research*, vol. 1, p. 311. (London: Newman).

85 Kesson, C. M. and Ireland, J. T. (1976). Phenformin compared with fenfluramine in the treatment of obese diabetic patients. *Practitioner*, **216** (1295), 577

86 Jenkins, D. J. A., Wolever, T. M. S., Hockaday, T. D. R. and Leeds, A. R. (1977). Treatment of diabetes with guar gum. *Lancet*, **ii,** 779

87 Kannel, W. B. and Gordon, J. (1974). Obesity and cardiovascular disease. The Framingham study. In W. L. Burland, P. Samuel and J. Yudkin (eds.). *Obesity*, p. 24. (London: Churchill Livingstone)

88 Keys, A. (1970). Coronary heart disease in seven countries. *Am. Heart Assoc. Monograph*, No. 29

89 Oliver, M. F. (1976). Dietary cholesterol, plasma, cholesterol and coronary heart disease. *Br. Heart J.*, **38,** 214

90 Miller, G. T. and Miller, N. E. (1975). Plasma high-density lipoprotein concentration and development of ischaemic heart disease. *Lancet*, **1,** 16

91 Gordon, T., Castelli, W. P., Hjortland, M. C., Kannel, W. B. and Dawber, T. R. (1977). High-density lipoproteins as a protective factor against coronary heart disease: The Framingham Study. *Am. J. Med.*, **62,** 707

92 Logan, R. L., Thomson, M., Riemersma, R. A., Oliver, M. F., Olsson, A. G., Rossner, S., Callmer, E., Walldios, G., Kaijser, L., Carlson, L. A., Lockerbie, L. and Lutz, W. (1978). Risk factors for ischaemic heart disease in normal men aged 40. *Lancet*, **1,** 949

93 Oliver, M. F. (1978). Diet and coronary heart disease. In J. Yudkin (ed.). *Diet of Man: Needs and Wants*, p. 69. (London: Applied Science)

94 Blum, C. B., Levy, R. I., Eisenberg, S., Hall, M., Goebel, R. H. and Berman, M. (1977). High density lipoprotein metabolism in man. *J. Clin. Invest.*, **60,** 795

95 Yudkin, J. (1972). Sucrose and cardiovascular disease. *Proc. Nutr. Soc.*, **31,** 331

96 Medical Research Council (1970). Report to the Medical Research Council by the working party on the relationship between dietary sugar intake and arterial disease. *Lancet*, **2,** 1265

97 Keys, A. (1973). Sucrose in the diet and coronary heart disease. *Atherosclerosis*, **18,** 352

98 Morris, J. N., Marr, J. W. and Clayton, D. G. (1977). Diet and heart: a postscript. *Br. Med. J.*, **2,** 1307

99 Raymond, T. L., Connor, W. E., Lin, D. S., Warner, S., Fry, M. C. and Connor, S. L. (1977). The interaction of dietary fibres and cholesterol upon the plasma lipids and lipoproteins, sterol balance and bowel function in human subjects. *J. Clin. Invest.*, **60,** 1429

100 Dept. of Health and Social Security (1974). *Diet and Coronary Heart Disease.* (London: HMSO)

101 Report of the Working Party of the Royal College of Physicians of London and the British Cardiac Society (1976). Prevent of coronary heart disease. *J. Roy. Coll. Phys. Lond.*, **10,** 213

102 Tyroler, H. A., Heyden, S. and Hames, C. G. (1975). Weight and hypertension: Evans county study of blacks and whites. In O. Paul (ed.). *Epidemiology and Control of Hypertension*, p. 177. (New York: Stratton)

103 Dahl, L. K. (1972). Salt and hypertension. *Am. J. Clin. Nutr.*, **25,** 231

104 Ramsay, L. E., Ramsay, M. H., Hettiarachchi, J., Davies, D. L. and Winchester, J. (1978). Weight reduction in a blood pressure clinic. *Br. Med. J.*, **2,** 244

105 Salel, A. F., Riggs, K., Mason, D. T., Amsterdam, E. A. and Zelis, R. (1974). The importance of type IV hyperlipoproteinaemia as a predisposing factor in coronary artery disease. *Am. J. Med.*, **57,** 897

106 Blacket, R. B., Woodhill, J. M., Leelarthaepin, B. and Palmer, A. J. (1975). Type IV hyperlipidaemia and weight gain after maturity. *Lancet*, **1,** 517

107 Nestel, P. and Goldrick, B. (1976). Obesity: changes in lipid metabolism and the role of insulin. In M. J. Albrink (ed.). *Clinics in Endocrinology and Metabolism – Obesity*, p. 53. (Philadelphia: Saunders)

108 Beaumont, J. L., Carlson, L. A., Cooper, G. R., Fejfar, Z., Frederickson, D. S. and Strasser, T. (1970). Classification of hyperlipidaemias and hyperlipoproteinaemias. *Bull. W. H. O.*, **43,** 8

109 Levy, R. I., Frederickson, D. S., Shulman, R., Bilheimer, D. W., Breslow, J. L., Stone, N. J., Lux, S. E., Sloan, H. R., Krauss, R. M. and Herbert, P. N. (1972). Dietary and drug treatment of primary hyperlipoproteinaemia, *Ann. Int. Med.*, **77,** 267

110 Carlson, L. A. and Olsson, A. G. (1975). Hyperlipidaemia and its management, In M. F. Oliver (ed.). *Modern Trends in Cardiology*, vol. 3, p. 405. (London: Butterworths)

3

Control of feeding and the psycho-pharmacology of anorexic drugs

J. E. Blundell and S. L. Burridge

DRUGS, OBESITY AND FEEDING

If pharmacological agents have a role in the treatment of obesity then their efficacy must be considered in the light of information about the systems controlling feeding behaviour and the mechanisms involved in the aetiology of obesity. In the past most pharmacological research relevant to obesity has been directed toward the development of anorexic drugs – appetite suppressants – on the understanding that a primary cause of obesity was the overeating which resulted from an excessive hunger[1]. Accordingly, the most obvious way to counter obesity was by drugs which inhibited hunger. However, the relationship between hunger, overeating and obesity is far from simple and it is widely recognized that human obesity does not arise from a single causal factor. Moreover, certain of the conditions important for the development of obesity may exist beyond the generally recognized boundaries of a physiological system and within the domain of psychological interactions. It follows that there is no simple policy available to guide the development of drugs to treat obesity, and one researcher has referred to the use of drugs in obesity as tantamount to quackery[2]. Indeed, it must be admitted that the overall advantage to weight loss brought about by drug administration is often small[3]. Consequently, these issues raise a number of questions regarding the use of drugs for the treatment of obesity:

(a) What should be the primary objective of pharmacological treatment – restriction of food intake or loss of body weight?
(b) Should different drugs be prescribed for different types of fat people whose condition may arise from quite different causal processes?
(c) Should drugs be administered as the sole form of treatment?

Further understanding of the potential efficacy of drugs in the treatment

53

The Treatment of Obesity

of obesity may be gained by considering the way in which drugs could interact with mechanisms controlling food intake and energy expenditure.

CONCEPTUALIZATION OF THE FEEDING PROCESS: PHARMACOLOGICAL APPROACHES

It is generally recognized that a system exists to regulate body weight in which metabolic, neural, and hormonal signals are integrated into a cohesive pattern. The basic elements of such a system are set out in Figure 1, which illustrates the interrelationship between behavioural and physiological processes. This system shows how post-ingestional signals, together with metabolic signals arising from the processing of nutrients, may be brought together to provide the basis of a link between central and peripheral mechanisms. It follows that disorders of this regulatory system may arise at a number of locations, and that therapeutic agencies may be directed at these sites. For example, the common (but inaccurate) belief that fat people experience excessive hunger may be counteracted by psychotherapeutic or behavioural strategies directed to point A. The

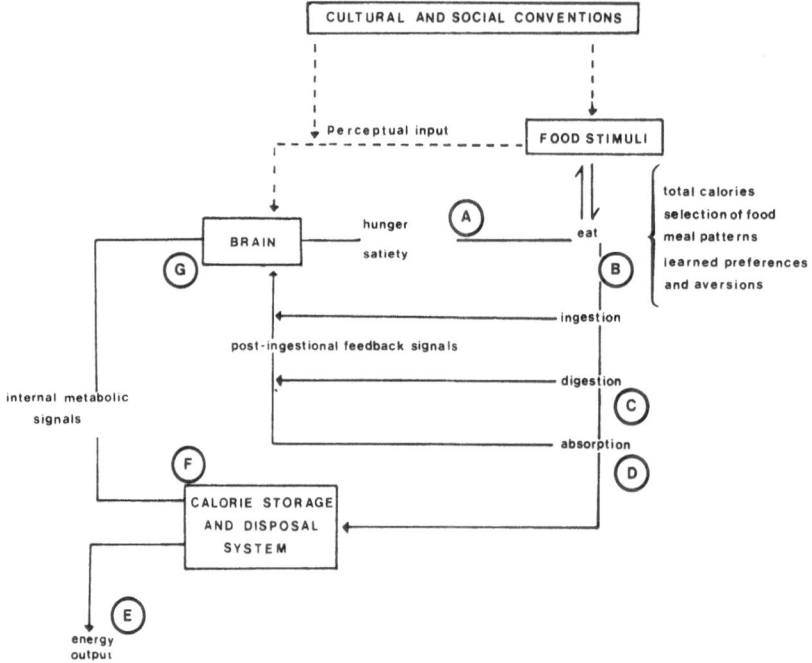

Figure 1 Working conceptualization of the system which functions to match food intake to energy requirements. The bold letters refer to points in the system toward which therapeutic techniques may be directed

process of eating (point B) may be constrained in a mild way by adherence to calorie-controlled diets or more severely by enforced starvation or jaw-clamping by means of a dental splint. The process of digestion may be directly inhibited by gastro-plasty which effectively reduces the volume of the stomach (point C) while absorption of nutrients can be obstructed by ileo-jejunum bypass operation (point D). In turn, the basal metabolic rate or energy output may be increased by a regime of physical exercise (point E), and there are instances of cosmetic surgery being carried out to directly remove adipose tissue (point F). More dramatically, brain surgery (point G) has been performed in an attempt to destroy central mechanisms giving rise to hunger motivation. In addition to these non-pharmacological techniques, attention has been drawn to the way in which drugs may perform similar functions[4] and the available pharmacological data have recently been reviewed[5].

The most widespread form of pharmacological treatment includes drugs designed to suppress food consumption (point B) by some action which is believed to inhibit hunger or enhance satiety (point A). The mechanisms through which such drugs are presumed to act will be discussed later. In addition drugs could act elsewhere in the system. For example, drugs acting on digestive activities or modifying the physicochemical characteristics of the stomach (point C) may hinder the processing of ingested nutrients and may have repercussions upon the act of feeding itself. The compound ($\pm$)-transepoxyaconitic acid is known to slow the rate of gastric emptying and to reduce food consumption in rats. In addition, inhibitors of pancreatic α-amylase can effectively reduce the bio-availability of carbohydrate by preventing the digestion of starch to maltose and consequently diminishing the amount of glucose available for absorption. Indeed, the strategy of interfering with nutrient absorption (point D) suggests a powerful route by which pharmacological agents could be used in the treatment of obesity. Various compounds satisfy the theoretical principles, including neomycin and cholestryramine which partially obstruct the absorption of fat, and perfluoroctyl bromide which reduces general nutrient absorption by providing an inert film of material over the stomach and intestines.

Among the compounds which may act at point F to inhibit lipid synthesis the most thoroughly researched is ($-$)-hydroxycitrate[6]. In rats this agent has been shown to reduce circulating levels of triglycerides and cholesterol and to reduce body weight[7]. Finally, considerable research is currently being devoted to the development of thermogenic drugs which increase basal metabolic rate (point E). Well-known agents such as dinitrophenol or the thyroid hormones do increase heat production and metabolic rate, but are not suitable for long-term therapeutic use.

It is clear that pharmacological agents, as well as non-pharmacological techniques, are theoretically capable of providing a treatment for obesity by intervening at various critical stages in the system regulating body weight. Further research will undoubtedly give rise to new pharmacotherapeutic tools. However, at the present time the standard form of pharmacological treatment of obesity is the inhibition of food intake, and it is worth examining how these agents interact with the physiological system regulating energy balance.

GENERAL CHARACTERISTICS OF ANOREXIC DRUGS

Many pharmacological agents are capable of reducing food intake but the term anorectic drug is usually applied only to that group of compounds which have been developed and marketed for the treatment of obesity. These drugs are usually assumed to exert their action by a suppression of appetite – the subjective experience of a desire to eat – and to act upon mechanisms controlling ingestion. However, these assumptions are often based upon scant and inadequate evidence. It may be questioned whether or not anorectic drugs intervene in the natural system which normally matches food intake to nutritional requirements, or whether feeding is simply obstructed by some vicarious action of the drug. The resolution of this problem depends on the design of animal and human experiments which can distinguish between the two possibilities.

The chemical structures of some of the more widely used anorexic drugs are illustrated in Figure 2. Many (not not all) of these drugs can be considered as elaborations of a basic β-phenylethylamine nucleus. However, subtle alterations in the physical structure of a drug may lead to striking changes in the physiological or behavioural effects that it induces[8]. For example, amphetamine itself is characterized by a number of well-documented effects including *inter-alia* anorexic action, central stimulant properties, mood enhancement, cardiovascular changes and a selective effect on certain neural transmitter agents (particularly the catecholamines). It is now generally considered that when amphetamine is administered clinically this constellation of effects leads to anorexia being associated with a number of bodily and psychological changes which provide a rationale for misuse of the drug or which give rise to the development of drug-dependence.

However, certain changes in the ring, side-chain or amino structure of amphetamine may lead to marked modification of the properties of the drug. For example, introducing a halogen group into the ring (as in chlorphentermine or fenfluramine), or forming a cylindrical structure in the side-chain (as in phenmetrazine) may lead to marked diminution in central stimulation and cardiovascular activity with little effect upon anorexic

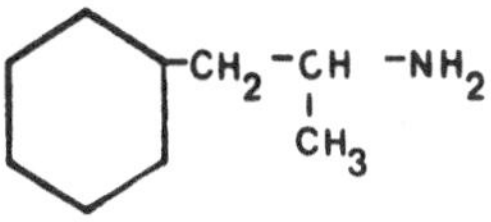

Amphetamine

BENZEDRINE; DUROPHET

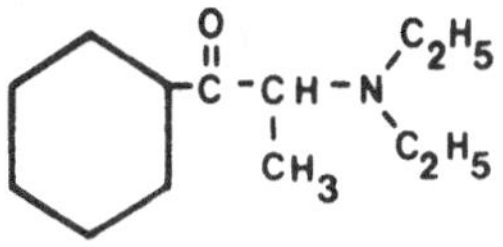

Diethypropion

TENUATE; APISATE

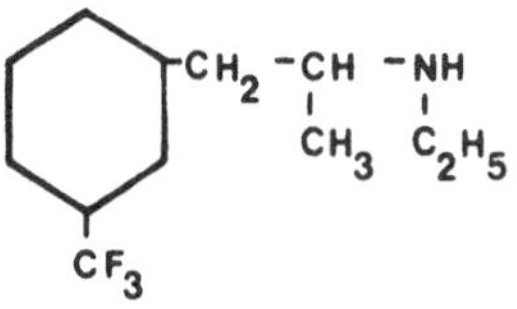

Fenfluramine

PONDIMIN; PONDERAX

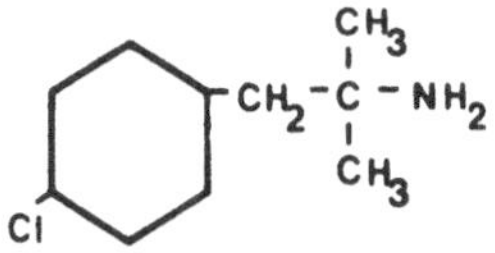

Chlorphentermine

PRESATE; LUCOFEN

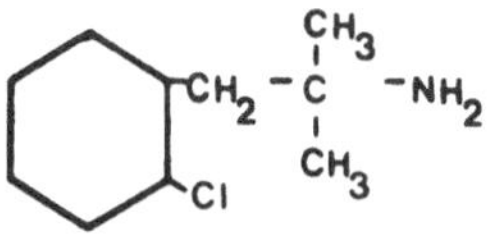

Clortermine

VORANIL

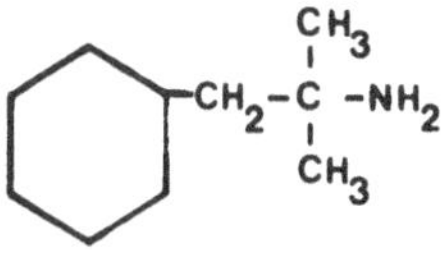

Phentermine

DUROMIN; IONAMIN

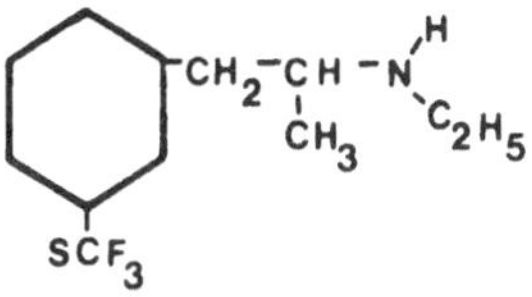

Tiflorex

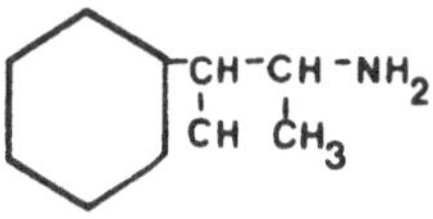

Phenylpropanolamine

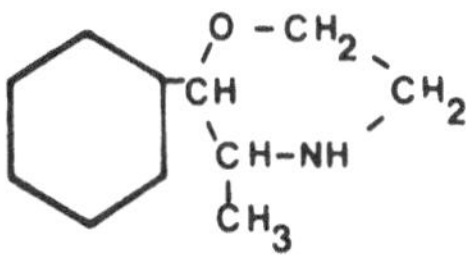

Phenmetrazine

PRELUDIN

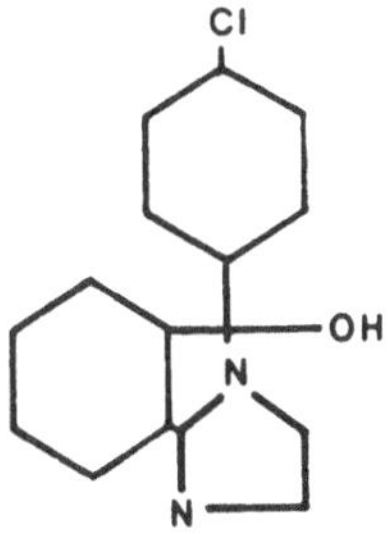

Mazindol

SANOREX; TERONAC

Figure 2 Structures of some drugs used in the treatment of obesity and for the experimental investigation of feeding. The trade name of the drug, where appropriate, is given in capitals potency. In addition, the drug may now exert a quite different action upon neurotransmitters. Consequently it is misleading to assume behavioural properties of drugs by considering their gross structure. For example, despite the superficial resemblance between fenfluramine and amphetamine, fenfluramine appears to have fewer properties in common with amphetamine than does mazindol which is structurally quite different[9]. At the moment a number of non-phenylethylamine compounds are being developed[5] and a close examination of the properties of these drugs will provide interesting data on the mode of action of anorectic agents.

CENTRAL AND PERIPHERAL MECHANISMS

Inspection of the variety of anorectic compounds (Figure 2) prompts a consideration of where they may act within the system regulating feeding–energy relationships (Figure 1). Some naturally occurring agents such as cholecystokinin[10] and glycerol[11] can inhibit feeding and reduce body weight in animals. It follows that synthetic anorexic compounds may act peripherally by adjusting the availability of these agents or of other metabolites. In particular, it has been suggested that certain drugs intervene directly in carbohydrate or lipid metabolisms and considerable attention has been focussed upon the activity of fenfluramine.

There are strong logical and empirical reasons for believing that the availability of glucose is one factor controlling nutritional intake[12]. This notion is embodied in the well-known glucostatic hypothesis of feeding. It has been reported that fenfluramine increases glucose uptake by muscle tissue *in vivo*[13] and exerts a hypoglycaemic action in normal, obese and diabetic subjects. *In vitro* studies using isolated human skeletal muscle or rat diaphragm have demonstrated that fenfluramine can significantly increase glucose uptake in the presence of insulin[14,15]. These studies have provided empirical support for the alleged 'glycoliptic' action of fenfluramine which incorporates the idea that its therapeutic action depends on the promotion of tissue uptake of glucose with a consequent decline in the availability of glucose for the synthesis and maintenance of lipid stores. However the glycoliptic action of fenfluramine has not found universal support[16], and there is no direct evidence to show that the action of fenfluramine on glucose metabolism is related either to weight loss or to a reduction in food consumption. It should be mentioned that other drugs notably, mazindol and tiflorex, also increase glucose uptake *in vitro*[17].

Certain studies have also demonstrated an effect of anti-obesity drugs on lipid metabolism. For example, fenfluramine given to human volunteers has been shown to increase plasma levels of free fatty acids, glycerol and ketone bodies and to reduce levels of triglycerides and total plasma lipids[18].

In addition, fenfluramine has been reported to decrease fat absorption from the diet[19], to reduce triglyceride synthesis in the liver[20] and to inhibit glycerol phosphate incorporation into lipids[21]. These data suggest that fenfluramine may slow lipid synthesis and increase the rate of fat breakdown. Similar evidence is available for the drug (−)-hydroxycitrate which inhibits fatty acid synthesis and reduces blood levels of cholesterol and triglycerides[6].

In addition to these effects on glucose and lipid metabolism drugs may also interfere with food consumption or fat synthesis at alternative peripheral sites (Figure 1). Fenfluramine has been reported to improve glucose tolerance by inhibiting gastric emptying following glucose administration[22] and to delay intestinal transit time[23]. These actions may contribute to the weight loss brought about by fenfluramine since it has been reported that the anti-obesity action of (±)-transepoxyaconitate depends upon a reduction in food intake which, in turn, is related to a reduction in the rate of gastric emptying[5].

For compounds such as (−)-hydroxycitrate and (±)-transepoxyaconitate, which probably do not enter the brain, the primary source of their anti-obesity action must be sought in peripheral mechanisms, though of course the consequences of these peripheral actions (changes in signals of gastric distension or alterations in blood concentrations of fat metabolites) are likely to be mediated via the central nervous system. However, all of the drugs shown in Figure 2 are believed to enter the brain readily, and current research favours the idea that their major actions are mediated by primary effects on the brain.

CNS MECHANISMS AND FEEDING –
THE CHANGING SCENE

The foundations of the role of CNS mechanisms in feeding were established when dramatic effects on food consumption and body weight were brought about by experimental manipulation of the hypothalamus using the stereotaxic procedure in the 1940s and 1950s. Various experiments demonstrated that damage to the ventro-medial zone of the hypothalamus gave rise to hyperphagia and obesity, while lateral hypothalamic damage caused aphagia and severe loss of body weight. This formed the basis of the classical dual-mechanism theory of the control of food intake, which emphasized the separation of zones in the hypothalamus and established the idea of distinct hunger and satiety centres[24]. This hypothesis offered a satisfactory answer for many of the questions regarding the stopping and starting of feeding. However, the mass of research which it stimulated revealed that the brain is not so simply organized. It is now recognized that

the dual-centre model requires to be radically revised[25]. There is of course
no doubt that experimental interventions in the lateral and ventro-medial
zones of the hypothalamus do produce striking effects upon food consumption and body weight – the real issue concerns the interpretation of
these effects. Although it is generally agreed that the hypothalamus must
be assigned a prominent role in the initiation, maintenance and termination
of food intake, it is no longer possible to sustain the idea that it contains
simple 'on' and 'off' biological devices. The revision of beliefs about the role
of the hypothalamus in feeding have been largely brought about by
neuropharmacological investigations. The introduction of techniques for
identifying neurochemical pathways in the brain, together with the
development of pharmacological tools for intervening selectively in neurochemical metabolism, has permitted a more sophisticated partitioning of
brain processes than that which has been provided in the past by the use of
electrical brain stimulation or non-specific electrolytic or electrothermal
lesioning techniques. The beginning of the neurochemical era of feeding
research, which dates from Grossman's introduction of direct chemical
stimulation of the brain, set in motion a research effort which has produced information to update the ideas generated by the earlier neuroanatomical era of research. The *zeitgeist* of the present decade has directed
the attention of researchers to the neurochemical basis of feeding and has
provided a rationale for beginning to understand the action of anorexic
drugs on food intake.

NEUROCHEMISTRY AND FEEDING

Information about the relationship between brain neurotransmitters and
feeding has arisen predominantly from three strategies: direct chemical
stimulation of specific brain loci, selective destruction of particular neurochemical pathways by means of a lesion or injected neurotoxin, and selective pharmacological manipulation of neurotransmitter metabolism. Over
the last few years most attention has been directed to the role of the
monoamines – particularly noradrenaline, dopamine and more recently
serotonin – although it is generally understood that alterations in a number
of other putative transmitter systems will exert some influence over
feeding activities.

Direct chemical stimulation of the brain
The idea of neurochemical coding for feeding behaviour was prompted
by the early studies of Grossman[26,27] indicating that local application of
the neurotransmitter noradrenaline (biologically active 1-isomer) through
a permanently indwelling hypothalamic cannula could induce a pro-

nounced bout of eating. Although Grossman's original work drew attention to the potency of exogenously administered noradrenaline it did not provide direct information about the function of endogenous noradrenaline. However, the involvement of endogenous noradrenaline was established by the administration of drugs which exert an indirect action upon transmitter functions. Thus desmethylimipramine – a drug believed to block the re-uptake of noradrenaline from the synaptic cleft – will potentiate eating in food-deprived rats[28]. This suggests that natural (deprivation-induced) feeding is accompanied by the release of noradrenaline from endogenous stores and that eating may be enhanced by drugs which facilitate this process or which prolong the action of noradrenaline after release. Indeed, experiments using a push–pull cannula technique have reported that food restriction is associated with the release of noradrenaline from the anterior hypothalamus[29]. Moreover, it has been established that the eating response to noradrenaline can be reduced by prior administration of an alpha-adrenergic blocking drug such as phentolamine but not by a beta-blocker such as propranolol[30]. A number of studies have confirmed that the site of action of the alpha-adrenergic feeding effect is around the paraventricular nucleus of the anterior hypothalamus[30-32]. On the other hand direct chemical stimulation at a slightly posterior site in the hypothalamus – around the peri-fornical region – will inhibit feeding behaviour[33]. In contrast to the adrenergic induction of feeding, this suppressive effect can be countered by drugs which are believed to block beta-adrenergic or dopamine receptors. Accordingly, it now appears that there are two separate sites within the hypothalamus which are pharmacologically distinguishable and which have opposite effects on eating[34]. However, these two sites do not correspond to the former division of the hypothalamus into lateral and ventro-medial zones.

Lesion studies and pharmacological intervention

Although it has been known for many years that there existed an uneven distribution of amines in the brain, histochemical procedures developed during the 1960s made it possible to map the detailed localization of the cell bodies, axons and terminals of noradrenaline, dopamine and serotonin[35]. Knowledge about these specific chemical pathways has not only helped to explain the dramatic involvement of certain hypothalamic zones in feeding, but has also necessitated a reappraisal of the nature of brain mechanisms controlling food intake[36,37].

For example, lesion studies using specific neurotoxins have revealed that an aphagic syndrome, similar to that seen after lateral hypothalamic lesions, can be brought about by the interruption of dopamine pathways of the nigro-striatal tract[38,39] or by the depletion of forebrain dopamine and noradrenaline[40]. Although effects observed after damage to the nigro-

striatal bundle are not identical with the effects seen after lateral hypothalamic lesions[41], these data are in keeping with the view that certain of the
consequences of large hypothalamic lesions are due to the interruption of
fibres of passage rather than to the destruction of specialized cell bodies[42].

The arrangement of fibre pathways shown in Figure 3 suggests that the

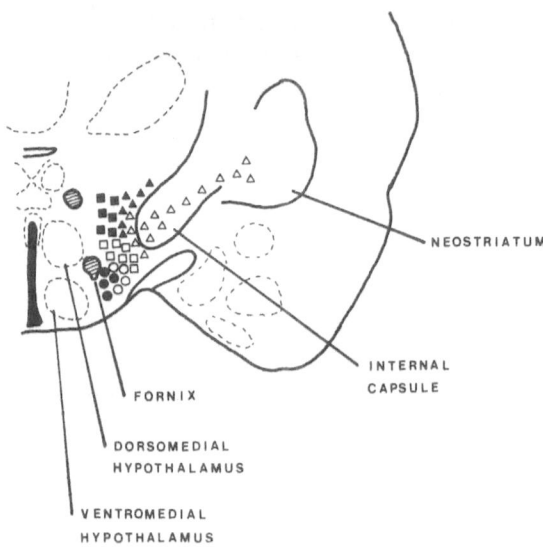

▲ MESO-LIMBIC DOPAMINE SYSTEM

△ NIGRO-STRIATAL SYSTEM

■ DORSAL NORADRENERGIC BUNDLE

□ VENTRAL NORADRENERGIC BUNDLE

● MEDIAL SEROTONERGIC SYSTEM

○ LATERAL SEROTONERGIC SYSTEM

NEOSTRIATUM

INTERNAL
CAPSULE

FORNIX

DORSOMEDIAL
HYPOTHALAMUS

VENTROMEDIAL
HYPOTHALAMUS

Figure 3 Cross-section of a ventral quadrant of rat brain showing the arrangement of chemical pathways in the lateral hypothalamic portion of the medial
forebrain bundle. (After Morgane[108])

behavioural and physiological effects of damage in the lateral hypothalamic
region will be critically dependent upon the extent of destruction in
particular amine systems. Moreover, in drawing attention to the role of
dopamine systems in the effects of lateral hypothalamic lesions the pharmacological approach has revealed that the deficits are not restricted to feeding
activities. Following lateral hypothalamic lesions and damage to the nigro-
striatal tract there are profound behavioural and physiological disturbances
resulting in widespread loss of abilities. These findings question the whole
concept that lateral hypothalamic lesions reveal important direct information about the control of food intake, and that there is a direct role for
dopamine systems in the overall regulation of energy balance.

It has also been suggested that certain amine pathways may be implicated in ventro-medial hyperphagia in a similar fashion to the involvement of dopamine fibre tracts in lateral hypothalamic aphagia. It appears that hyperphagia and weight gain do not occur when small lesions in the medial hypothalamus are restricted to the ventro-medial nucleus itself but only if the tissue surrounding that nucleus is damaged[43]. This is consistent with the report that hyperphagia and obesity can result from micro-knife cutting of tissue immediately behind the ventro-medial nucleus[36]. Further work combining coronal knife cuts with electrolytic lesions and with para-saggital knife cuts has strongly suggested that the hyperphagia resulting from damage to the medial hypothalamus depends upon the interruption of fibres passing adjacent to the ventro-medial nucleus.

Although these reports implicate a projection system in hypothalamic hyperphagia they do not identify the particular pathway. However when the neurotoxin 6-hydroxydopamine is injected directly into the ventral noradrenergic pathway (but not the dorsal pathway) rats begin overeating and become obese[44,45]. This pathway arises in the pons largely from cell groups labelled A1, A2, A5 and A9, and passes rostrally to provide dense innervation in the thalamus and hypothalamus. It follows that the ventral noradrenergic bundle could be the pathway involved in medial hypo-thalamic hyperphagia. Moreover, it has been reported that the destruction of a ventral noradrenergic tegmental projection abolishes the suppression of eating brought about by certain injections into the perifornical hypo-thalamus. However, these pharmacological experiments cannot as yet fully account for medial hypothalamic hyperphagia.

Although most research has focussed upon the role of the catecholamines (noradrenaline and dopamine) in feeding, the indoleamine serotonin may also be involved (Figure 3). In general, agents or procedures that enhance the synaptic activity of serotonin bring about an inhibition of food intake, whereas procedures which diminish or block synaptic activity lead to over-eating, weight gain, and in some cases, even to obesity[46]. In particular, it has been reported that intraventricular injections of parachlorophenyl-alanine, which inhibit the synthesis of serotonin, may give rise to hyper-phagia and obesity[47] whilst specific damage to the median raphe nuclei (B8) gives rise to a noticeable weight increase. Since the degeneration of serotonin tracts following raphe lesions counteract medial hypothalamic hyperphagia, serotonin mechanisms may be involved in the ventro-medial syndrome.

Although a precise role for serotonin has not been established, it seems possible that it may exert a general inhibitory effect on feeding[48], act as a secondary satiety system, provide day and night control of satiety pro-cesses, or modulate other systems controlling body weight (see Ref. 48). In addition, recent research has demonstrated how a serotonin mechanism could control the selection of protein taken in the diet[49,50].

This mechanism depends on a process which regulates the transport of tryptophan (a precursor of serotonin) from the blood into the brain, and provides exciting possibilities for interpreting the relationship between brain chemistry and feeding.

Conceptualization of the interaction of amines in the control of feeding

In considering neurochemical mechanisms and feeding it is important to maintain a sense of proportion. It is difficult to attempt to conceptualize brain-behaviour processes without reducing the extreme complexity of the brain to naive simplicity. However, Figure 4 illustrates a possible working

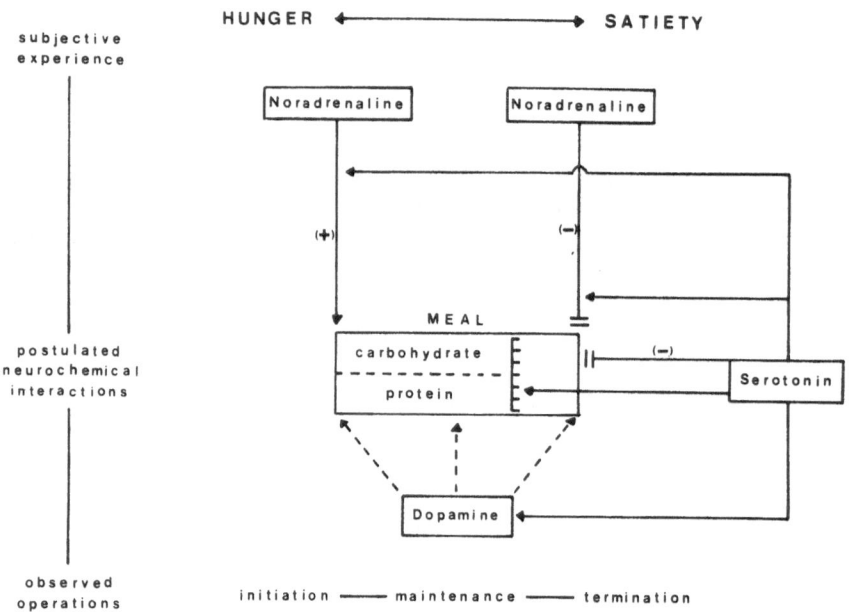

Figure 4 Working conceptualization of the possible roles of monoamine neurotransmitters in feeding, based on current evidence, illustrating how manipulations of these amine systems influence food consumption

conceptualization of brain chemistry and feeding on the basis of current research developments. The figure displays how noradrenaline, dopamine and serotonin systems could interact to control the moment-to-moment consumption of food and the selection of certain dietary components. It is clear from this model that experimental manipulation of any of these amines may give rise to changes in feeding, often in an unpredictable way. For example, both dopamine agonists and blockers may inhibit feeding[51,52], a finding which questions whether or not dopamine mechanisms intervene in the system which matches food intake to nutritional requirements. Instead it appears that dopamine plays an indirect role in feeding, possibly acting as a 'gate' to permit the expression of eating or by influencing the rate of the feeding process. Indeed, changes in dopamine metabolism may give rise to alterations in arousal and sensorimotor integration, resulting in general behavioural disturbances of which feeding impairments could represent one obvious example.

The suggested relationship between the neurotransmitters and feeding (Figure 4) needs to be regarded with some caution. First, a number of other brain chemicals such as acetylcholine, gamma-aminobutyric acid, and certain prostaglandins are known to influence food intake under various circumstances. Secondly, the model does not indicate the possible way whereby metabolic information is converted into neurochemical activity, nor the way in which changes in neurotransmitter systems become translated into behaviour. Thirdly, it is widely recognized that activities in the three major brain amine systems are interdependent. The neuroanatomical links between the differing clusters of cell bodies imply that at any moment in time the tendency to feed will be determined not by a single neurotransmitter system but by the prevailing neurochemical flux – the overall balance between the activities of a number of systems. The notion of a neurochemical flux may be difficult to grasp, but is probably fundamental to the understanding of the central action of anti-obesity agents.

PHARMACOLOGICAL MANIPULATION OF FEEDING: METHODOLOGICAL ISSUES

The purpose underlying the development of anti-obesity drugs should be the design of pharmacological agents which intervene in the natural regulatory system which normally matches food intake to nutritional requirements. Although anorexic drugs with differing pharmacological profiles may intervene selectively in this natural system a full understanding of the mechanisms of action is often hindered by the use of insensitive procedures for measuring feeding activities. It is very easy to disturb feeding in animals and humans by a pharmacological challenge. The central issue is to determine whether such a drug-induced inhibition of eating really represents a non-specific blockade or behaviour, or results from a specific physiological change within the regulatory system.

Anorexic drug testing

Typically, in the research development of anorexic drugs the usual measurement of food intake is derived from drug screening procedures and consists of weighing the amount of food consumed by animals[53] (usually rats) during a discrete test interval (usually 1 or 2 h) following a period of food deprivation. Alternatively, animals may be placed on cyclic training programmes when they are obliged to eat at specific times during the day when allowed access to food. These techniques have arisen since anorexic drugs are developed as a commercial exercise rather than for the convenience of theoretical biology, and the pharmaceutical industry demands screening procedures which can be administered rapidly and simply. There are reasons for believing that these procedures are not effective either for producing precise information about anorexic drug action or for throwing light upon the processes controlling food intake.

First, the weight of food consumed in a discrete interval of time may conceal information about the manner in which the anorexic drug inhibited food consumption; for example, an animal may fail to eat because of competing or interfering activities. Indeed it now seems likely that a good deal of the inhibitory action of high doses of $(+)$-amphetamine on food intake can be accounted for by the inability of animals to eat due to stereotypy or to excessive hyperactivity. Moreover, the single measure of weight of food consumed fails to indicate whether a drug is acting to inhibit the onset of eating, to slow the process of eating or to hinder its execution, or to prematurely terminate an eating episode.

Secondly, although brief periods of eating following long periods of deprivation are typical for drug experiments they are not typical of animal or human behaviour and are not usually encountered in natural animal (or human) feeding repertoires. Consequently, it is possible that drugs are being evaluated under highly abnormal circumstances[54]. Thirdly, it is known that food deprivation can modify brain neurotransmitter systems. It follows that drugs administered to severely deprived animals may be intervening in atypical brain metabolism.

In summary, the combined use of severe deprivation periods and short food tests represent a procedure which may be highly insensitive to certain drug effects, may create circumstances for abnormal behaviour and which may modify drug action in an unknown way by altering brain chemistry.

Food intake and feeding behaviour

Certain of the defects mentioned above can be overcome by distinguishing between food intake and feeding behaviour. Many experiments in this research field have been based on the concept of a homeostatic system regulating body weight. In these circumstances, it is appropriate for experimenters to regard feeding activities as a means of supplying fuel to the internal system and the primary focus of attention becomes the total amount of food which is taken in. Feeding behaviour involves a complex interaction between internal physiological processes and the structural and psychological conditions of the environmental milieu. This interaction is displayed in the means of procuring food, the relative allocation of time and effort to feeding and other activities, the storing and preparation of food, the distribution of feeding throughout the day and to the actual manner of food consumption. Accordingly, feeding behaviour for animals and humans can best be viewed as a bio-physical interaction between the demands of the internal system and the demands of the habitat. It follows that experimental studies on drugs and feeding should be designed to enhance the ecological validity of the data.

One way of achieving this is to take into account the fact that mammalian food intake is a discontinuous process in which periods of eating alternate with non-eating. Freely feeding animals eat in discrete meals[55] and within meals short bouts of eating are separated by short episodes of other activities[56]. Accordingly, it is possible to measure feeding by assessing various parameters of meal patterns such as the number of meals taken over a given period, meal sizes, meal durations, inter-meal intervals and certain relationships among these variables such as the ration of meal size to pre- or post-meal interval[57]. In addition certain intra-meal characteristics may be assessed, such as the number, size and duration of eating bouts and the relationship between bouts of eating and non-eating activities[58]. These techniques draw attention to the distinction between food intake – usually assessed by measurement of weight of food consumed – and eating behaviour, assessed by close analysis of the pattern of the feeding response. Although measurement of the sheer bulk of food consumed may throw light upon regulatory mechanisms, it seems likely that a more detailed behavioural analysis will be required in order to determine the way in which brain processes exert a moment-to-moment control over feeding activities. Moreover, it has been proposed that only studies of the eating behaviour of freely-feeding animals provide data which illustrate how an animal is matched to its ecological niche[59].

Hunger and satiety

The particular technique used to measure feeding in any experimental situation is important, for the data are frequently used to establish whether changes have been brought about by alterations in 'hunger' or 'satiety'. These terms cannot be measured directly but may only be inferred indirectly from objective data. Both terms have high explanatory value and are generally assumed to refer to quite separate facets of the feeding process: hunger being reflected in a tendency to purposely seek out food and to initiate feeding, while saiety refers to the termination of food consumption resulting from the act of food ingestion itself. These definitions may tempt researchers to ascribe any changes in food intake to a modification of either hunger or satiety. However, it is often a moot issue whether animals and humans begin to eat because they have been overcome by hunger or because satiety has waned. Equally, eating may stop if hunger is suppressed or satiety enhanced. Although these terms are often used inadvisedly, their widespread occurrence throughout the literature suggests a reluctance to abandon their use in favour of purely operational descriptions of feeding. However, it should be recognized that before the labels 'hunger' and 'satiety' can be assigned to changes in feeding, the data must include more information than the crude weight of food consumed[60].

MECHANISMS OF ACTION OF ANOREXIC DRUGS

Although it is clear that certain anorexic drugs produce changes in peripheral metabolism (see the section 'Central and peripheral mechanism') current research favours the view that these drugs act via brain mechanisms controlling food intake. Now that the dual-centre view has been undermined, the mechanisms of action of anorexic drugs must be sought in neurochemical language (see Figure 4).

Despite some methodological shortcomings, certain clear statements . have emerged. First, most of the anorexic drugs which have been employed clinically, such as amphetamine, diethylpropion, mazindol and fenfluramine, produce dramatic effects on brain neurotransmitters – particularly the monoamines. Secondly, pharmacological and neurological manipulations which alter the activity of amines in the brain significantly adjust the potency of anorexic drugs to suppress food intake. Thirdly, different neurochemicals appear to be involved in the action of different drugs. In general, it appears that catecholamines play a dominant role in the actions of amphetamine, phentermine, mazindol and diethylpropion while the action of fenfluramine appears to be mediated via serotonergic systems. Accordingly, the neurochemical conceptualization of feeding control as set out in Figure 4 can provide a working framework for beginning to understand the mechanisms underlying anorexic drug action.

The puzzle of amphetamine
The methodological problems which hinder the interpretation of data derived from the pharmacological manipulation of feeding are exemplified in research on amphetamine. Although the idea that amphetamine has a suppressive effect on appetite was mooted more than 40 years ago[61], it is still an open question whether or not amphetamine exerts this effect through a mechanism related to the natural system linking food intake and

nutritional needs. The problem rests on the fact that amphetamine produces multiple physiological and behavioural effects including *inter alia* changes in heart rate, body temperature and bodily movements and postures. In animals low doses of amphetamine (less than 1·5 mg/kg) give rise to hypermotility, whilst higher doses induce a syndrome characterized by compulsive gnawing, licking and sniffing – this constellation of features is known as stereotypic behaviour. Carlton has proposed that amphetamine anorexia arises from the incompatibility of the eating response with the effects of the drug on locomotion[62], and Lyon and Robbins have also suggested that the effect of amphetamine on eating is secondary to more widespread effects of the drug on other behavioural systems[63]. In human research it could similarly be argued that the effect of amphetamine on appetite (or hunger) is due to conscious attention being diverted towards other physiological changes, or to the masking of hunger by an overwhelming awareness of other sensations. Consequently, it is possible that both in animal and human experiments the effect of amphetamine on eating may have little to do with *direct* action on a system regulating energy intake.

This issue can be more deeply examined by considering the effect of amphetamine on brain chemistry. There is good evidence that amphetamine exerts a dominant and primary effect on the release and uptake of the catecholamines – noradrenaline and dopamine – while producing apparently less important effects on indoleamine metabolism. However, the catecholamines are strongly implicated in other behavioural effects of amphetamine – particularly locomotor activity and stereotypy. For example, brain lesions which deplete forebrain noradrenaline attenuate amphetamine-induced locomotor activity[64], in a similar fashion to lesions of a part of the mesolimbic dopamine system. In addition there is widespread agreement that the nigro-striatal dopamine pathway is implicated in amphetamine-induced stereotypy. Consequently the problem can be summarized in the following statements:

1. Amphetamine gives rise to an inhibition of eating, to hyperactivity and stereotypy.
2. Amphetamine produces dramatic changes in the activity of noradrenaline and dopamine systems.
3. These transmitters are implicated in the manifestation of eating, locomotor activity and stereotypy.
4. Can the effects of amphetamine on eating be dissociated from its effects on motor activity and posture?

Support for a dissociation is provided by evidence that certain hypothalamic lesions can diminish the anorexic effect of amphetamine[65] without effect on amphetamine-induced arousal[66]. Moreover, micro-injections of amphetamine into the perifornical zone of the hypothalamus can inhibit eating while producing no obvious effects on activity[33]. However, these dissociations cannot easily be ascribed to an action upon separate neurotransmitter systems for amphetamine anorexia may be antagonized by either blockade of noradrenergic receptors[33,67] or by the disruption of brain dopamine systems[68,69]. The issue may be partly resolved by comparing the antagonistic effects of certain treatments at differing doses of amphetamine. This is a reasonable strategy for it is known that the behavioural effects seen after amphetamine injection are dose-related. Recently, two procedures have been used to counter the anorexic action of amphetamine: destruction of the ventral noradrenergic bundle and blockade of dopamine receptors by neuroleptics. Figure 5 is a composite diagram comprising data from separate experiments. It indicates that although both procedures antagonize amphetamine anorexia only the noradrenergic treatment achieves this effect at the lowest dose (0·5 mg/kg).

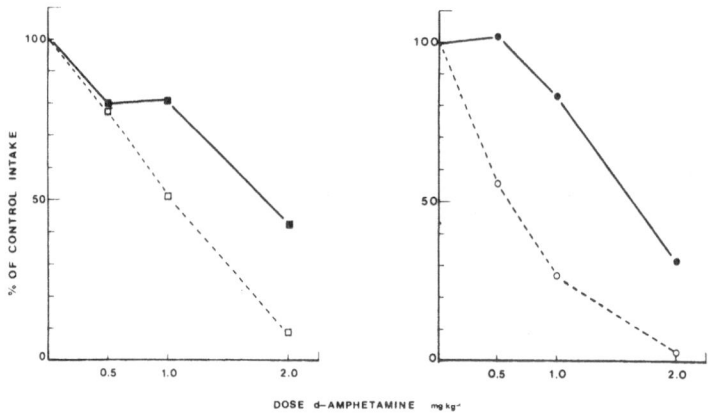

Figure 5 Effect of dopamine blockade and forebrain noradrenaline depletion on amphetamine anorexia. The left-hand graph shows the inhibition of food intake (1 h test) following amphetamine administration (open symbols) and after amphetamine plus dopamine receptor blockers (solid symbols). The results for the dopamine blockade represent pooled data from separate experiments using subanorectic doses of pimozide, spiroperidol, *cis*-(2)-flupenthixol and piflutixol (Burridge – unpublished data). The right-hand graph shows the suppression of food intake brought about by amphetamine administration in intact animals (open symbols) and in rats with experimentally induced depletion of brain noradrenaline (solid symbols). These data are taken from the experiments of Ahlskog[45] and Carey[64]

Consequently, it can be suggested that the inhibition of eating brought about by low doses of amphetamine is noradrenergically mediated while at higher doses dopamine systems become involved. It is tempting to conclude that a low dose of amphetamine may give rise to a pure anorexic response, while at higher doses of the drug the inhibition of eating is largely due to the occurrence of disruptive motor activity and stereotypy. This conceptualization of amphetamine's action is summarized in Figure 6 which shows the dose-related behavioural effects of amphetamine together with the postulated contribution of noradrenergic or dopaminergic systems.

However, this hypothesis only partially accounts for the action of amphetamine because recent reports have drawn attention to certain surprising paradoxical observations. When amphetamine has been administered to non-deprived animals, it has been observed that very low doses actually induce eating in rats[52] and mice[70]. These effects are reminiscent of a similar action of amphetamine in rats[71] and cats[72] recovering from the effects of lateral hypothalamic lesions. These findings clearly show that any drug effects must be related to the state of the animal and to environmental variables[73].

Certain of these unexpected effects of amphetamine only become apparent under testing regimes which depart from the standard technique of weighing the food consumed by deprived animals. Indeed it is worth drawing attention to one further paradoxical effect which could only have been detected by examining the microstructure of the feeding process. This has revealed that while amphetamine may decrease the amount of food consumed by an animal, it can actually increase the rate at which eating occurs[52].

The mechanism of amphetamine anorexia has been considered at length since amphetamine has been regarded as a reference drug in pharmacological research on feeding. The findings reveal how little is really known about the way in which amphetamine suppresses eating, and suggests that the effects of amphetamine in animals and man should be interpreted cautiously. Similar strictures naturally apply to drugs which share some of the behavioural and neurochemical properties of amphetamine.

The fenfluramine story

Although there appears to be only a slight structural difference between amphetamine and fenfluramine (Figure 2) this molecular alteration gives rise to marked neurochemical, pharmacological and behavioural differences. Unlike amphetamine, fenfluramine does not produce hyperactivity or stereotypy, and consequently there may be fewer methodological problems surrounding an interpretation of its anorexic action. Moreover, unlike amphetamine, fenfluramine appears to have little effect on brain catecholamines but produces a long-lasting depletion of brain serotonin. In addition, fenfluramine facilitates the release of serotonin and blocks its re-uptake[74]. One obvious interpretation of these findings is that the anorexic effect of fenfluramine is mediated via a serotonergic, rather than a catecholaminergic, mechanism.

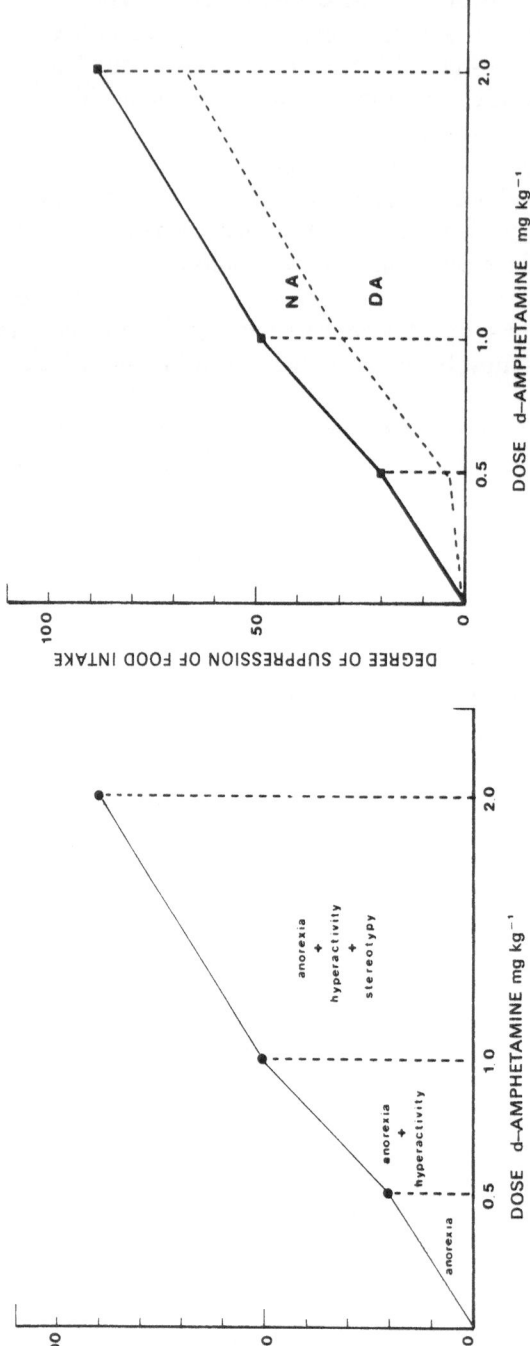

Figure 6 Summary model to demonstrate the dose-related effects of amphetamine. The left-hand graph shows the changes in observed behaviour with increasing doses of amphetamine and illustrates that with higher doses of amphetamine disturbing changes could contribute to the inhibition of food consumption. The right-hand graph shows the postulated contribution of noradrenergic and dopaminergic systems to the observed behavioural effects

Because of its novel combination of behavioural and neurochemical properties, fenfluramine is a drug of considerable theoretical importance. First, the absence of any marked behavioural arousal (sedation is more common) illustrated that it was possible to induce anorexia pharmacologically without increasing CNS activation. Secondly, the fairly selective neurochemical action of fenfluramine drew attention to the possible involvement of serotonin in feeding.

This has been evaluated by various studies designed to assess the anorexic effect of fenfluramine in conjunction with procedures believed to block or disrupt the functioning of serotonin system. For example, the anorexic action of fenfluramine can be partially countered by injections of serotonin receptor-blocking drugs such as methysergide[75], methergoline[76], cinanserin[77] and cyproheptadine[74]. In addition, pretreatment of rats with intraventricular injections of 5,6-dihydroxytryptamine – a neurotoxin which destroys serotonin terminals – has been shown to attenuate the anorexic effect of fenfluramine[78], although contradictory results have been obtained[69]. However, the most striking reduction of fenfluramine's anorexic effect has been achieved following electrolytic lesions of the median raphe nuclei[79], though it should be noted that other studies have shown lesser effects of this procedure[80] or no effect at all[64,81]. The overall equivocal nature of these results probably arises from the complex way in which brain serotonin systems influence feeding and the relatively crude techniques used for intervening in brain serotonin metabolism.

The general principle which has emerged is that those procedures which counter amphetamine anorexia have little effect on fenfluramine or may even enhance its action, while procedures which antagonize fenfluramine anorexia have little or no effect on the action of amphetamine. The anorexic action of the two drugs can be dissociated not only by these pharmacological techniques but also by intrahypothalamic injections[82], hypothalamic lesions[83] and by simultaneous administration of a serotonin precursor[84]. It is necessary to emphasize the consistent differences between amphetamine and fenfluramine on every test model which has been employed, for the separation of the effects of the drugs suggests that they exert an effect on food consumption through quite distinct mechanisms and modes of action. Furthermore, investigations of the micro- and macrostructure of feeding have suggested that amphetamine and fenfluramine exert quite distinct influences over the eating process[52,85]. On the one hand amphetamine seems to block the onset of eating but accelerates the rate of consumption, whereas fenfluramine brings eating to a premature termination while slowing the rate of consumption. It may be useful to characterize those differences as an effect of amphetamine on hunger and an action of fenfluramine on satiety[86].

Summary

The detailed discussion of mechanism of action has been limited to amphetamine and fenfluramine, since the bulk of research on anorexic drugs has been carried out on these two compounds. It is clear that these two drugs exert quite distinct profiles of action on brain chemistry and behaviour. It appears that they adjust different components of the system which controls the feeding process. At present, the most plausible explanation for these different adjustments is obtained by referring to the neurochemical effects of the drugs. Drugs which display a prominent effect on catecholamines will share behavioural properties with amphetamine, while drugs acting on brain serotonin may resemble a fenfluramine pattern. Among the more frequently used anorexic compounds (Figure 2), phentermine, diethylpropion and mazindol probably act via catecholamine mechanisms, but it is not clear which agents, apart from fenfluramine, act via serotonin[87].

ANOREXIC DRUGS: EXPERIMENTAL STUDIES IN MAN

The previous section has shown that although anorexic compounds reduce food consumption in animals (under certain conditions) the mechanisms of action are not fully understood. The real test of the depth of understanding of drug action arises when data from animal studies are compared with data from experiments in man. Clinical studies have shown that over short periods of time anorexic compounds may produce significant reduction in body weight compared with placebo treatment. It may be questioned whether or not this results from a capacity of the drug to pharmacologically influence the system controlling food consumption in response to nutritional requirements.

In order to investigate this, it is necessary to assess the effect of drugs upon a number of factors, including subjective experience, motivation and behaviour. An examination of subjective experience will reveal the extent and quality of those changes induced by the drug which are accessible to the subject's conscious awareness. Measurement of motivation will show the extent to which the drug has manipulated the subject's willingness to begin eating and the disposition to actively acquire food. A close inspection of actual eating behaviour will indicate the capacity of the drug to suppress food consumption or to adjust the manner in which consumption takes place. Ideally, the anorexic drug should diminish the subjective appreciation of appetite, suppress the disposition to initiate eating and reduce the amount of food consumed. Although it might be expected that these three elements always co-vary, in fact, they can be dissociated under particular circumstances. Accordingly, it is not intuitively obvious how anorexic drugs inhibit feeding in humans.

Subjective sensations induced by drugs are frequently measured by check lists or rating scales, and this technique has revealed that a number of drugs including amphetamine[88], phentermine[89], diethylpropion[90], mazindol[91], fenfluramine[92] and tiflorex[93] can reduce the subjective appreciation of hunger or appetite. However, a number of studies have detected a paradoxical failure of some drugs to produce an alteration in subjectively perceived appetite[94] despite changes in body weight[95]. Moreover, in certain cases, drugs have produced changes in hunger ratings only when explicitly identified as appetite depressants[96]. Although one study with amphetamine has observed a weak correlation between the effects of the drug on food intake and appetite[88], a recent investigation has reported the absence of any systematic relationship between ratings of hunger and the amount of food consumed[97]. In a further study with fenfluramine, a high dose markedly reduced hunger ratings in female subjects but gave rise to a small increase in the amount of food eaten[92]. Taken together, these findings indicate that subjective ratings of appetite or hunger do not invariably provide a reliable index of the effectiveness of the drug to inhibit food intake or to reduce body weight.

The lack of certainty and poor predictive value of some of the available data draws attention to the methodological difficulties of measuring appetite. Simple rating scales are widely used in experimental studies and clinical trials to assess the effectiveness of anorexic drugs. The fundamental problem arises from a lack of understanding of the mental processes which takes place when people are requested to report their feelings of hunger in an experimental setting. This may present the subject with an entirely novel intellectual task, for although people frequently refer to 'hunger' in casual conversation, the reference is usually vague and few people clearly recognize the origins of the feelings to which the term hunger is attributed. It is clear that for many people the subjective search for the stimuli which lead to a verbal statement of hunger constitutes a difficult task. Indeed, what are the appropriate and relevant target stimuli to which people should refer when assessing the intensity of hunger? Do the stimuli reside in the physiological domain as sensations in the mouth and throat, the viscera or the limbs; or do they exist in the psychological domain as feelings of light-headedness, dizziness or irritability? Alternatively, some people may simply relate hunger to the interval of time which has elapsed since their last meal. It follows that it may be difficult to assess the effectiveness of anorexic drugs by means of subjective ratings of hunger; for if people are not normally consciously aware of the sensations which give rise to hunger, they may be led into error when attempting to identify the significance of adjustments induced by a drug.

Because of these methodological difficulties, alternative techniques have been considered for measuring hunger motivation. For example, it has been suggested that the degree of salivation elicited by a palatable food (conditioned salivation) is a reliable predictor of the amount of food likely to be consumed[98]. Moreover, it has been reported that amphetamine significantly reduced conditioned salivation even though the drug produced no effect on hunger rating[99]. Accordingly, it is possible that conditioned salivation may provide a sensitive non-verbal index of hunger motivation.

The most convincing illustration of the efficacy of an anorexic drug will be reduction in food consumption. However, a crude measure of the amount of food consumed gives as little information about the mechanism of action of anorexic drugs in man as it does in animals. Accordingly, various techniques have been designed to provide continuous and detailed information about feeding during single or multiple meals. For example, fine measurement has been achieved by the use of liquid food dispensers[100,101]; automated solid food sandwich dispensers[93] and through the analysis of video-taped recordings of meals[97]. Pudel's work on the time-relationships of eating has established the identity of biological satiety curves – the rate of eating of normal-weight subjects diminishing as the meal progresses. On the other hand, the intake curves for obese subjects are usually linear in form. Although this monitoring technique can differentiate the rate of eating of normal-weight and obese subjects, the data from drug experiments are more difficult to understand. In a cleverly designed study fenfluramine was given to obese, latent obese and non-obese subjects and tablets were clearly labelled as appetite suppressants or placebo. However, a quarter of the fenfluramine tablets were labelled as placebo. All three groups were found to reduce their food intake at lunch in their own homes by about 30% regardless of the tablet contents, as long as they were marked as an appetite suppressant. But when fed in the laboratory from a food-dispensing machine neither the label nor the drug affected the food intake of the obese groups, although normal-weight subjects reduced calorie intake by some 23% on fenfluramine.

A recent study, using techniques developed in animal studies, has compared the action of amphetamine and fenfluramine on the selection of and preference for particular foods, and on the microstructure of eating[97]. Although both drugs suppressed the weight of food consumed to an equal degree, clear differences between the drugs emerged on the finer measures of eating. For example, amphetamine delayed the onset of the meal and shortened the duration of the meal but actually increased the rate at which food was loaded into the mouth by reducing the pauses between mouthfuls. On the other hand, fenfluramine slowed the pace of consumption by reducing the rate of chewing. In addition, amphetamine significantly decreased the amount of protein consumed during the meal and reduced preference for high-protein foods, while fenfluramine had no marked effect on these parameters. These findings are quite consistent with data from animal studies, and demonstrate that these two compounds exert noticeably different actions upon the feeding process.

At present, there is no understanding in depth of the mechanism of drug-induced anorexia in man. It is necessary to recognize that subjective appetite and food consumption are far more complex processes than has been hitherto apparent and that the elucidation of the mechanism of action of drugs upon these processes will require more sophisticated procedures than rating scales and food weighings. A major influence on research has been the limitation of experimental design by non-scientific considerations in order to publicly demonstrate the efficacy of a drug through its power to lower hunger ratings, rather than to examine the mechanism through which the drug may displace feelings of hunger and obstruct eating. The understanding of the mechanism of anorexic drugs is confronted by the difficulty in knowing whether subjects who inspect their psychological and physiological domains to make decisions about the level of appetite and the likelihood of initiating eating are actually responding to changes relevant to their nutritional status or to vicarious actions of the drugs which divert attention toward distracting side-effects. However, certain studies which have widely sampled subjective feelings and closely monitored behavioural changes do suggest that drugs with distinct pharmacological profiles do intervene differently in the processes which control feelings of hunger and eating behaviour in man.

IMPLICATIONS OF CURRENT RESEARCH

This chapter has reviewed current knowledge about the mode of action of certain anorexic drugs and about the way in which they interact with other factors which influence food consumption. It seems appropriate to try to relate this information to a better understanding of how drugs may be used in the treatment of obesity.

It is clear that the effect of anorexic drugs is dependent upon the nature of the prevailing conditions. For example, in animal studies, the effectiveness of a drug depends upon the physiological state of the animal and upon the quality of available foodstuff, while in humans, it depends on the beliefs of the subject and upon the setting in which feeding takes place. This means that in addition to the pharmacological action of the drug, many other factors affect food consumption. In the doses in which they are prescribed, drugs are a fairly mild form of therapy when compared with treatments such as dental wiring, metabolic starvation and bypass surgery.

There is no doubt that drugs could more effectively suppress food intake if they were administered in doses sufficient to cause a massive adjustment to the interval system similar to that produced by major abdominal surgery. However the circumstances under which drugs are taken means that the drug must not only intervene in a biological system but must also act in such a way as to out-manoeuvre the socio-cultural variables which tend to resist any change in feeding habits. Because feeding is controlled both by internal and external stimuli, drugs probably act only upon a small portion of the total feeding domain. Consequently, even if a particular drug did produce a clear and continuing reduction in hunger, external constraints and long-term habits to do with the buying, preparation and consumption of specific foods may be sufficiently powerful to overcome the effect of the drug. For this reason it has been suggested that anorexic drugs could be administered in conjunction with techniques of behaviour therapy designed to deal with the demands of the psychological and social environment[102]. In this way the two therapies could provide conjoint control over the internal and external milieux. Moreover, the drug would be acting in a setting which complemented its action rather than in a situation which opposed its efficacy. So far this clinical approach has been adopted in two studies known to the authors. One short study in which phentermine was combined with a behavioural programme for 8 weeks showed no advantage for the conjoint treatment[103], while a 6-month study of fenfluramine together with behaviour modification produced a significantly greater weight loss than the behavioural treatment alone[104].

Secondly, it is known that obese people differ from each other in terms of their aetiology and that anorexic drugs represent a heterogeneous cluster of compounds. Accordingly, while certain drugs may be effective for some people they may be useless for others. One advancement in the pharmacotherapy of obesity would be to develop a method for tailoring the drug treatment to the individual's requirements. For example, since drugs may differ in their capacity to inhibit the initiation of eating, to bring eating to a halt, or to adjust the microstructure of feeding, then drugs with differing modes of action could be administered to obese people with differing feeding profiles. More particularly, since it has been argued that some obese individuals display manifest hunger[105], while others lack an ability to stop consumption once eating has begun[106] then drugs with specific pharmacological profiles could be discriminately prescribed to counter hunger or to promote satiety.

The practice of administering drugs in conjunction with a dietary schedule of low-calorie foods is not new. However, those studies which have drawn attention to the intimate relationship between dietary composition and brain chemistry suggest that it may be possible to use dietary control in a more subtle and rational manner. For example, the effectiveness of drugs acting via serotonin systems could theoretically be intensified by administering a diet rich in tryptophan (a precursor of serotonin).

Naturally such regimes should be carried out cautiously to ensure that undesirable changes do not occur in other behavioural domains also influenced by serotonin fluctuations.

It is likely that within the next few years new pharmacological treatments will become available and would be embraced within new therapeutic strategies guiding the administration of drugs. Recognition of the complex interactive processes influencing the final outcome of drug administration draws attention to the importance of adopting a realistic framework to guide the use of drugs. Perhaps drugs for the treatment of obesity can be used to give patients the opportunity to learn something about themselves rather than to bring about an automatic restriction of food consumption. Whatever programme is taken up for the treatment of obesity, patients will always have to feed, and feeding is an activity which links the biological domains of energy transactions with the psychological domain of knowledge. Consequently, in experimental settings drugs can be used as tools to further explore the processes underlying the control of hunger and feeding, while in the clinic drugs could be used as tools to permit patients to better understand the forces – biological and psychological – which control their lives.

References

1 Blundell, J. E. (1977a). Hunger and satiety in the control of food intake: implications for the treatment of obesity. *La Clinica Dietologica*, **4,** 3

2 Bruch, H. (1973). *Eating Disorders: Obesity, Anorexia Nervosa and the Person Within*. (New York: Basic Books)

3 Scoville, B. A. (1976). Review of amphetamine-like drugs by the Food and Drug Administration: Clinical data and value judgements. In G. A. Bray, (ed.), *Obesity in Perspective*, p. 441. (Washington, DC: US Government Printing Office)

4 Blundell, J. E. (1975). Anorexic drugs, food intake and the study of obesity. *Nutrition (Lond.)*, **29,** 5

5 Sullivan, A. C. and Comai, K. (1978). Pharmacological treatment of obesity. *Int. J. Ob.* (In press)

6 Sullivan, A. C., Triscari, J., Hamilton, J. G. and Miller, O. N. (1974). Effect of (−)-hydroxycitrate upon the accumulation of lipid in the rat. II. Appetite. *Lipids*, **9,** 129

7 Sullivan, A. C., Triscari, J. and Speigel, H. E. (1977). Metabolic regulation as a control for lipid disorders. II. Influence of (−)-hydroxycitrate on genetically and experimentally induced hypertriglyceridemia in the rat. *Am. J. Clin. Nutr.*, **30,** 777

8 Biel, J. H. (1970). Structure–activity relationships of amphetamine and derivatives. In E. Costa and S. Garattini (eds.), *Amphetamine and Related Compounds*, p.3. (New York: Raven Press)

9 Garattini, S. and Samanin, R. (1976). Anorectic drugs and neurotransmitters. In T. Silverstone (ed.), *Food Intake and Appetite*, p.82. (Berlin: Dahlem Konferenzen)

10 Antin, J., Gibbs, J., Holt, J., Young, R. C. and Smith, G. P. (1975). Cholecystokinin elicits the complete behavioural sequence of satiety in rats. *J. Comp. Physiol. Psychol.*, **89,** 784

11 Wirtshafter, D. and Davis, J. D. (1977). Body weight: reduction by long-term glycerol treatment. *Science*, **198**, 1271

12 Le Magnen, J. (1976). Interactions of glucostatic and lipostatic mechanisms in the regulatory control of feeding. In D. Novin, W. Wyrwicka and G. Bray (eds.), *Hunger: Basic Mechanisms and Clinical Implications*, p.89. (New York: Raven Press)

13 Butterfield, W. J. H. and Whichelow, M. J. (1968). Fenfluramine and muscle glucose uptake in man. *Lancet*, **2**, 109

14 Kirby, M. J. and Turner, P. (1974). Effect of fenfluramine and norfenfluramine on glucose uptake by the isolated rat diaphragm. *Br. J. Pharmacol.*, **50**, 477

15 Kirby, M. J. and Turner, P. (1975). Fenfluramine and norfenfluramine on glucose uptake into skeletal muscle. *Postgrad. Med. J.*, **51**, (Suppl. 1), 73

16 Garrow, J. S., Belton, E. A. and Daniels, A. (1972). A controlled investigation of the 'Glycoliptic' action of fenfluramine. *Lancet*, **2**, 559

17 Turner, P. and Kirby, M. J. (1977). Some evidence for a peripheral mechanism of action of some anti-obesity drugs. Presented at 2nd Int. Cong. Obesity, October 23–26, Washington

18 Pawan, G.L.S. (1969). The effect of fenfluramine on blood lipids. *Lancet*, **1**, 498

19 Bizzi, A. Venerone, E. and Garattini, S. (1973). Effect of fenfluramine on the intestinal absorption of triglycerides. *Eur. J. Pharmacol.*, **23**, 131

20 Kaye, J. P., Tomlin, S. and Galton, D. J. (1975). The effect of fenfluramine and its derivatives on triglyceride secretion by the liver of the rabbit. *Postgrad. Med. J.*, **51** (Suppl. 1), 95

21 Brindley, D. N. and Bowley, M. (1975). Effects of fenfluramine and related compounds on the synthesis of glycerolipid by rat liver. *Postgrad. Med. J.*, **51**, 91

22 Page, M. G., Morville, M. and Corkey, B. E. (1977). Fenfluramine-mediated improvements in glucose tolerance: comparison with phenformin. Presented at 2nd. Int. Cong. Obesity, October 23–26, Washington

23 Le Dourec, J. (1963). The taking of food – a physiological study. Ph.D. thesis. Faculty of Pharmacology, University of Paris

24 Stellar, E. (1976). The CNS and appetite: historical introduction. In T. Silverstone (ed.) *Appetite and Food Intake*, p.15. (Berlin: Dahlem Konferenzen)

25 Blundell, J. E. (1976a). The CNS and feeding. In T. Silverstone (ed.), *Appetite and Food Intake*, pp.109–128. (Berlin: Dahlem Konferenzen)

26 Grossman, S. P. (1960). Eating or drinking elicited by direct adrenergic or cholinergic stimulation of hypothalamus. *Science*, **132**, 301

27 Grossman, S. P. (1962). Direct adrenergic and cholinergic stimulation of hypothalamic mechanisms. *Am. J. Physiol.*, **202**, 872

28 Montgomery, R. B., Singer, G., Purcell, A. T., Narbeth, J. and Bolt, A. C. (1971). The effects of intrahypothalamic injections of desmethylimipramine on food and water intake of the rat. *Psychopharmacol.*, **19**, 81

29 Gugten, J. V., De Kloet, E. R., Versteeg, D. H. G. and Slangen, J. L. (1977). Regional hypothalamic catecholamine metabolism and food intake in the rat. *Brain Res.*, **135**, 325

30 Leibowitz, S. F. (1975a). Ingestion in the satiated rat: role of alpha and beta receptors in mediating effects of hypothalamic adrenergic stimulation. *Physiol. Behav.*, **14**, 743

31 Booth, D. A. (1967). Localisation of the adrenergic feeding system in the rat diencephalon. *Science*, **158**, 515

32 Davis, J. R. and Keesey, R. E. (1971). Norepinephrine-induced eating; its hypothalamic locus and an alternative interpretation of action. *J. Comp. Physiol. Psychol.*, **77**, 394

33 Leibowitz, S. F. (1975b). Amphetamine: possible site and mode of action for producing anorexia in the rat. *Brain Res.*, **84**, 160

34 Leibowitz, S. F. (1976). Brain catecholaminergic mechanisms for control of hunger. In D. Novin, W. Wyrwicka, and G. Bray (eds.). *Hunger: Basic Mechanisms and Clinical Implications*, p.1. (New York: Raven Press)

35 Falck, B. (1962). Observations of the possibilities of the cellular localisation of monoamines by a fluorescence method. *Acta Physiol. Scand.*, **56** (Suppl. 197), 1

36 Grossman, S. P. (1975). Role of the hypothalamus in the regulation of food and water intake. *Psychol. Rev.*, **82**, 200

37 Myers, R. D. (1975). Brain mechanisms in the control of feeding: a new neurochemical profile theory. *Pharmacol. Biochem. Behav.*, **3**, (Suppl. 1), 75

38 Ungerstedt, U. (1971). Adipsia and aphagia after 6-hydroxydopamine induced degeneration of the nigro-striatal dopamine system. *Acta Physiol. Scand.*, (Suppl. 367), 95

39 Marshall, J. F., Richardson, J. S. and Teitelbaum, P. (1974). Nigro-striatal bundle damage and the lateral hypothalamic syndrome. *J. Comp. Physiol. Psychol.*, **87**, 800

40 Zigmond, M. J. and Stricker, E. M. (1973). Recovery of feeding and drinking by rats after intraventricular 6-hydroxydopamine and lateral hypothalamic lesions. *Science*, **182**, 717

41 Marshall, J. F. (1976). Neurochemistry of central monoamine systems as related to food intake. In T. Silverstone (ed.). *Appetite and Food Intake*, p.43. (Berlin: Dahlem Konferenzen)

42 Morgane, P. J. (1961). Alterations in feeding and drinking behaviour of rats with lesions of globi pallidi. *Am. J. Physiol.*, **201**, 420

43 Gold, R. M. (1973). Hypothalamic obesity: the myth of the ventromedial nucleus. *Science*, **182**, 488

44 Ahlskog, J. E. and Hoebel, B. G. (1973). Overeating and obesity from damage to a noradrenergic system in the brain. *Science*, **182**, 166

45 Ahlskog, J. E. (1974). Food intake and amphetamine anorexia after selective forebrain norepinephrine loss. *Brain Res.*, **82**, 211

46 Blundell, J. E. (1977b). Is there a role for serotonin (5-hydroxy-tryptamine) in feeding? *Int. J. Ob.*, **1**, 15

47 Breisch, S. F., Zemlan, F. P. and Hoebel, B. G. (1976). Hyperphagia and obesity following serotonin depletion by intraventricular parachlorophenyl-alanine. *Science*, **192**, 382

48 Blundell, J. E. (1978). Serotonin and feeding. In W. B. Essman and L. Valzelli (eds.), *Serotonin in Health and Disease*. (New York: Spectrum Publications, Inc.) (In press)

49 Ashley, D. V. and Anderson, G. H. (1978). Decrease in protein but not energy intake in the self-selecting rat. *J. Neurochem.* (In press)

50 Wurtman, R. J. and Fernstrom. J. D. (1974). Effect of the diet on brain neurotransmitters. *Nutr. Rev.*, **32**, 193

51 Heffner, T. G., Zigmond, M. J. and Stricker, E. M. (1977). Effects of dopaminergic agonists and antagonists on feeding in intact and 6-hydroxydopamine treated rats. *J. Pharmacol. Exp. Ther.*, **201**, 386

52 Blundell, J. E. and Latham, C. J. (1978a). Pharmacological manipulation of

feeding: possible influences of serotonin and dopamine on food intake. In R. Samanin and S. Garattini (eds.). *Central Mechanisms of Anorectic Drugs.* (New York: Raven Press). (In press)

53 Tedeschi, D. H. (1966). Pharmacological evaluation of anorectic drugs. In P. Mantegazza and R. Piccinini (eds.). *Methods in Drug Evaluation,* p. 341. (Amsterdam: North Holland)

54 Moran, G. (1975). Severe food deprivation: some thoughts regarding its exclusive use. *Psychol. Bull.,* **82,** 543

55 Richter, C. P. (1927). Animal behaviour and internal drives. *Quart. Rev. Biol.,* **2,** 307

56 Wiepkema, P. R. (1971a). Behavioural factors in the regulation of food intake. *Proc. Nutr. Soc.,* **30,** 142

57 Le Magnen, J. and Tallon, S. (1966). La periodicitée spontanée de la prise d'aliments ad libitum du rat blanc. *J. Physiol.* (Paris), **58,** 323

58 Wiepkema, P. R. (1971b). Positive feedbacks at work during feeding. *Behaviour,* **39,** 266

59 Collier, G., Hirsch, E. and Hamlin, P. H. (1972). The ecological determinants of reinforcement in the rat. *Physiol. Behav.,* **9,** 705

60 Blundell, J. E. and Latham, C. J. (1978b). Pharmacology of food and water intake. In S. Cooper and K. Brown (eds). *Chemical Influences on Behaviour.* (London: Academic Press) (In press)

61 Nathanson, M. H. (1937). The central action of beta-aminopropyl-benzene (Benzedrine). *J. Am. Med. Assoc.,* **108,** 528

62 Carlton, P. (1963). Cholinergic mechanisms in the control of behaviour by the brain. *Psychol. Rev.,* **70,** 19

63 Lyon, M. and Robbins, T. (1975). The action of central nervous system stimulant drugs: A general theory concerning amphetamine effects. In W. B. Essman and L. Valzelli (eds.). *Current Developments in Psychopharmacology,* vol. 2. (New York: Spectrum Publications, Inc.)

64 Carey, R. J. (1976). Effects of selective forebrain depletions of norepinephrine and serotonin on the activity and food intake effects of amphetamine and fenfluramine. *Pharmacol. Biochem. Behav.,* **5,** 519

65 Blundell, J. E. and Leshem, M. B. (1974). Central action of anorexic agents: effects of amphetamine and fenfluramine in rats with lateral hypothalamic lesions. *Eur. J. Pharmacol.,* **28,** 81

66 Campbell, B. A. and Baez, L. A. (1974). Dissociation of arousal and regulatory behaviour following lesions of the lateral hypothalamus. *J. Comp. Physiol. Psychol.,* **87,** 142

67 Frey, H. H. and Schultz, R. (1973). On the central mediation of anorexigenic drug effects. *Biochem. Pharmacol.,* **22,** 3041

68 Carey, R. J. and Goodall, E. B. (1975). Alteration of amphetamine anorexia by unilateral nigro-striatal lesions. *Neuropharmacol.,* **14,** 827

69 Hollister, A. S., Ervin, G. N., Cooper, B. R. and Breese, G. (1975). The roles of monoamine neural systems in the anorexia induced by (+)-amphetamine and related compounds. *Neuropharmacol.,* **14,** 715

70 Dobrzanski, S. and Doggett, N. S. (1976). The effects of (+)-amphetamine and fenfluramine on feeding in starved and satiated mice. *Psychopharmacol.,* **48,** 283

71 Stricker, E. M. and Zigmond, M. J. (1976). Recovery of function following damage to central catecholamine containing neurons: A neurochemical model for the lateral hypothalamic syndrome. In J. M. Sprague and A. N. Epstein

(eds.). *Progress in Psychobiology and Physiological Psychology*, p. 121. (New York: Academic Press)

72 Wolgin, D. L., Cytawa, J. and Teitelbaum, P. (1976). The role of activation in the regulation of food intake. In D. Novin, W. Wyrwicka and G. Bray (eds.). *Hunger: Basic Mechanisms and Clinical Implications*, p.179. (New York: Raven Press)

73 Antleman, S. M. and Caggiula, A. R. (1977). Norepinephrine–dopamine interactions and behaviour. *Science*, **195**, 646

74 Garattini, S., Bonaccorsi, A., Jori, A. and Samanin, R. (1974). Appetite suppressant drugs: past, present and future. In L. Lasagna (ed.). *Obesity: Causes, Consequences and Treatments*, p.70 (New York: Medoom Press)

75 Blundell, J. E., Latham, C. J. and Leshem, M. B. (1973). Biphasic action of a 5-hydroxytryptamine inhibitor on fenfluramine-induced anorexia. *J. Pharm. Pharmacol.*, **25**, 492

76 Jesperson, J. and Scheel-Kruger, J. (1973). Evidence for a difference in mechanism of action between fenfluramine and amphetamine-induced anorexia. *J. Pharm. Pharmacol.*, **25**, 49

77 Clineschmidt, B. V. (1973). 5,6-dihydroxytryptamine: suppression of anorexigenic effect of fenfluramine. *Eur. J. Pharmacol.*, **24**, 405

78 Clineschmidt, B. V., McGuffin, C., and Werner, A. B. (1974). Role of monoamines in the anorexigenic actions of fenfluramine, amphetamine and p-chloromethamphetamine. *Eur. J. Pharmacol.*, **27**, 313

79 Samanin, R., Ghezzi, D., Valzelli, L. and Garattini, S. (1972). The effects of selective lesioning of brain serotonin or catecholamine containing neurons on the anorectic activity of fenfluramine and amphetamine. *Eur. J. Pharmacol.*, **19**, 318

80 Fuxe, K., Farnebo, L. O., Hamberger, B. and Ogren, S. O. (1975). On the 'in vivo' and 'in vitro' actions of fenfluramine and its derivatives on central monoamine neurons, and their relation to the anorectic action of fenfluramine. *Postgrad. Med. J.*, **51**, (Suppl. 1), 35

81 Sugrue, M. F., Goodlet, I. and McIndeward, I. (1975). Failure of depletion of rat brain serotonin to alter fenfluramine-induced anorexia. *J. Pharm. Pharmacol.*, **27**, 950

82 Blundell, J. E. and Leshem, M. B. (1973). Dissociation of the anorexic effects of fenfluramine and amphetamine following intra-hypothalamic injection. *Brit. J. Pharmacol.*, **47**, 183

83 Blundell, J. E. and Leshem, M. B. (1975a). Hypothalamic lesions and drug induced anorexia. *Postgrad. Med. J.*, **51**, (Suppl. 1), 45

84 Blundell, J. E. and Leshem, M. B. (1975b). Effect of 5-hydroxytryptophan on food intake and on the anorexic action of amphetamine and fenfluramine. *J. Pharm. Pharmacol.*, **27**, 31

85 Blundell, J. E. and Leshem, M. B. (1975c). Analysis of the mode of action of anorexic drugs. In A. Howard (ed.). *Recent Advances in Obesity Research*, Vol. 1. (London: Newman Press)

86 Blundell, J. E., Latham, C. J. and Lesham, M. B. (1976). Differences between the anorexic action of amphetamine and fenfluramine: possible effects on hunger and satiety. *J. Pharm. Pharmacol.*, **28**, 471

87 Garattini, S. (1978). Pharmacological agents and feeding. In G. Bray (ed.). *Recent Advances in Obesity Research 2.* (London: Newman Press) (In press)

88 Silverstone, J. T. and Stunkard, A. (1968). The anorectic effect of dexamphetamine sulphate. *Br. J. Pharmacol. Chemother.*, **33**, 513

89 Silverstone, J. T. (1972). The anorectic effect of a long-acting preparation of phentermine (Duromine). *Psychopharmacol.*, **25**, 315

90 Silverstone, J. T., Cooper, R. M. and Begg, R. R. (1970). A comparative trial of fenfluramine and diethylpropion in obesity. *Br. J. Clin. Prac.*, **24**, 423

91 Johnson, W. G. and Hughes, J. T. (1977). The evaluation of mazindol in the treatment of obesity. Presented at 2nd. Int. Cong. Obesity, October 23–26, Washington

92 Silverstone, A. J., Fincham, J. and Campbell, D. B. (1975). The anorectic activity of fenfluramine. *Postgrad. Med. J.*, **51** (Suppl. 1), 171

93 Fincham, J. and Silverstone, J. T. (1977). The anorectic effect of triflorex, a new appetite suppressant compound. Presented at 2nd. Int. Cong. Obesity, October 23–26, Washington

94 Kroger, W. S. (1962). A comparison of anorexigenic drugs in the treatment of the resistant obese patient. *Psychosomatics*, **3**, 454

95 Malcolm, A. D., Mace, P. M., Ontar, K. P. and Pawan, G. L. S. (1972). Experimental evaluation of anorexigenic agents in man: a pilot study. *Proc. Nutr. Soc.*, **31**, 12A

96 Penick, S. B. and Hinkle, L. E. Jr. (1964). The effect of expectation on response to phenmetrazine. *Psychosom. Med.*, **26**, 369

97 Rogers, P. J. and Blundell, J. E. (1978). Effect of anorectic drugs on food intake, hunger, food selection and the microstructure of eating in man. (Submitted for publication)

98 Wooley, S. C. and Wooley, O. W. (1973). Salivation to the sight and thought of food: a new measure of appetite, *Psychosom. Med.*, **35**, 136

99 Wooley, O. W., Wooley, S. C., Williams, B. S. and Nurre, C. (1977). Differential effects of amphetamine and fenfluramine on appetite for palatable food in humans. *Int. J. Ob.*, **1**, 293

100 Hoebel, B. G., Krauss, I. K., Cooper, J. and Willard, D. (1975). Body weight decreased in humans by phenylpropanolamine taken before meals. *Obesity and Bar. Med.*, **4**, 200

101 Pudel, J. E. and Oetting, M. (1977). Eating in the laboratory: behavioural aspects of the positive energy balance. *Intl. J. Ob.*, **1**, 369

102 Blundell, J. E. (1976b). Strategies and tactics in the use of anti-obesity drugs. *Lancet*, **2**, 804

103 Brightwell, D. R. and Sloan, C. L. (1978). Effects of a combined behavioural and pharmacologic programme on weight loss. Presented at 2nd. Int. Cong. Obesity. October 23–26, Washington

104 Craighead, L., O'Brien, R. and Stunkard, A. (1978). New treatments for Obesity. Paper read at the American Psychiatric Association meeting, May 8–10, Atlanta

105 Nisbett, R. E. (1972). Hunger, obesity and the ventromedial hypothalamus. *Psychol. Rev.*, **79**, 433

106 Stunkard, A. J. (1968). Environment and obesity: recent advances in our understanding of the regulation of food intake in man. *Fed. Proc.*, **27**, 1367

107 Morgane, P. J. (1975). Anatomical and neuro-biochemical bases of the central nervous system control of physiological regulations and behaviour. In G. Mogenson and F. Calaresu (eds.). *Neural Integration of Physiological Mechanisms and Behaviour*, p.24. (Toronto: University of Toronto Press)

4

Clinical use of anti-obsesity agents

J. F. Munro

INTRODUCTION

It has been estimated that well over 5 million prescriptions were written for the anti-obesity drugs in 1966 in the United Kingdom. Since then, the number of scripts issued has steadily fallen to 'only' slightly more than 3 million prescriptions in 1975. This figure would suggest that either the anti-obesity drugs are effective or that they are being extensively over-prescribed. At present, more than one-third of subjects enrolling in a slimming organization will have previously taken at least one anti-obesity agent, and more than three-quarters of subjects referred by general practitioners to a hospital obesity clinic will have previously received drug therapy. It follows that subjects with a weight problem of sufficient concern to make them seek medical attention may, at present, reasonably expect to be prescribed a weight-reducing drug. Certainly most general practitioners prescribe at least one anti-obesity agent, and the majority of patients say that they find such drugs are helpful. Indeed, in a recent survey undertaken by the Consumers' Association, appetite-suppressant drugs were rated by women slimmers to be the best method of achieving rapid weight loss. However, only 16% of these women considered that dieting with the aid of appetite-reducing pills was a successful method of producing a long-term weight loss[1].

In spite of drug treatment, many subjects seeking medical help will continue to have a weight problem, and in their case either the drugs are ineffective or they are only of short-term benefit, or they are not being used properly. In an attempt to resolve this dilemma, three questions must be considered

(i) do anti-obesity drugs produce significant weight loss?
(ii) what happens to this weight loss if and when the drug is discontinued?

(iii) what, if any, is the role of the present anti-obesity agents in the overall, long-term management of obesity?

In theory, a drug will promote weight loss either if it causes a subject to eat less, or if it reduces the available food consumed, or if it leads to an increase in energy expenditure. Although it is possible that the so-called appetite-suppressants may exert a significant anti-obesity effect by increasing the peripheral utilization of energy substrate, it is generally considered that they primarily act centrally as anorectic agents. Their mode of action has been fully described in the previous chapter. This chapter deals with the clinical aspects of the currently available anti-obesity drugs, dealing in turn with those acting principally through the catecholamine systems, those affecting the serotonergic systems and other drugs.

DRUGS ACTING ON CATECHOLAMINES

Amphetamine

Although amphetamine has been of considerable clinical and scientific interest since it was first synthesized in 1927, its weight-reducing properties were not immediately appreciated. It then became apparent that the amphetamines could produce variable but significant suppression of appetite in man, the effect being maximal after about 2 h. For many years they were widely prescribed as anti-obesity agents. However, there has been a major change in attitude towards their use since it was appreciated in the early 1960s that amphetamine abuse might be as serious a problem as opiate addiction, particularly in schoolchildren or young adults. For this reason, their use as anorectic agents has been banned in certain countries, including Sweden and Australia. In many other countries prescription is controlled. In the United Kingdom amphetamine and compounds containing amphetamine are covered by the 'Misuse of Drugs' Act 1971 and its regulations. In addition, the British Medical Association has recommended that practitioners voluntarily cease to prescribe such products in the management of obesity. It is unfortunate that they remain available as anorectic drugs. Certainly, although the amphetamines have been used as the yardstick against which other agents are evaluated, there is no evidence to suggest that amphetamine is significantly more effective than the alternative less stimulant phenylalanine derivatives. Although the individual risk of addiction in carefully selected patients may be low, the very availability of the drug leaves open the potential for grave misuse. In addition to its anorectic properties, it has been taken to produce euphoria or to overcome fatigue. Dependence may develop gradually and the chronic amphetamine misusers may appear remarkably normal even while taking large doses. Others may present with the features of a chronic anxiety state. The amphetamines also may cause a psychotic illness which may be difficult to distinguish from paranoid schizophrenia. If the drug can be successfully withdrawn, the psychotic symptoms settle within a few days, though withdrawal depression may be so severe as to cause suicide. Deaths can also occur from accidental or deliberate self-poisoning. Other side-effects of long-term administration include possible growth retardation in children and permanent brain damage in chronic abusers[2].

Amphetamine-containing compounds should never be prescribed in the management of obesity.

Phenmetrazine

Phenmetrazine has anorectic properties comparable to those of amphetamine. However, its side-effects are also similar to the parent compound. Given as an appetite-suppressant, its stimulant qualities may result in drug dependence. Like amphetamine, it has been extensively abused by the non-obese. It can cause a toxic psychosis, has been reported to produce permanent brain damage and is thought to be teratogenic[2]. Many countries, including the United Kingdom, apply the same restrictions on phenmetrazine-containing compounds as they use to control amphetamine. Although phenmetrazine may be somewhat less dangerous than amphetamine, there are no clinical situations in which its use can be justified.

Diethylpropion

Clinical pharmacology
Diethylpropion is another amphetamine analogue which has been used extensively since 1960. Little has been published about its absorption and fate in man. The acute administration of 50 mg of diethylpropion will produce significant reduction in hunger rating in non-obese male volunteers within 30 min of administration. The drug has no direct effect on carbohydrate metabolism, and it has been claimed that it produces anorexia without causing clinically significant stimulation of the central nervous system and that it has few sympathomimetic properties. Indeed, the intravenous administration of doses up to 10 mg of diethylpropion in patients with various forms of cardiac disease fail to produce significant changes in blood pressure, pulse rate or electrocardiogram.

Side-effects
Diethylpropion clearly exerts a sympathomimetic effect in some subjects, as reflected by the reported incidence of such side-effects as increased sweating, palpitations and dryness of the mouth. Likewise, the drug can cause stimulation of the central nervous system, as illustrated pharma-

cologically by its effect on critical flicker frequency and on rapid eye movement (REM) sleep and clinically by the reported incidence of restlessness, irritability, increased energy, euphoria and insomnia. Generally speaking, however, these effects are not unduly distressing though they may be experienced by up to a third of treated subjects. They rarely are of such severity as to necessitate discontinuation of treatment and the drug is a popular choice amongst patients themselves. Withdrawal depression is not a problem, and no cases of death from diethylpropion have been reported. As might be expected in any drug with some stimulant properties, abuse has occurred. A small number of female subjects have presented with diethylpropion psychosis. So far the reported cases have been restricted to subjects who have previously taken amphetamine and/or phenmetrazine. Clearly, diethylpropion should be avoided in patients known to have previously abused drugs and also patients with features suggesting a major personality disorder.

Efficacy

Diethylpropion has been widely prescribed for nearly 20 years and there are numerous double-blind studies which confirm that it will produce significantly greater weight loss than placebo. It has been suggested that 'tolerance' does not occur and that its weight-reducing properties will persist undiminished for as long as 6 months[3]. However, only seven patients taking the active preparation completed this particular study, and the design of the trial failed to take into consideration the influence of mean weight change on those subjects who defaulted. In contra-distinction, another study, with a similar defect in design, reported a plateauing of mean weight loss after 10 weeks of therapy and a mean weight gain occurred after 18 weeks until the end of the 24-week study period[4]. Certainly, the common experience is for substantial weight loss to occur only for a few weeks. This is illustrated on Table 1, which summarizes the results of three recent double-blind 12-week studies in which diethylpropion was compared with placebo therapy[5-7]. The mean weight losses achieved with diethylpropion were highly significant when compared with that obtained by placebo, but the sum of the mean weight loss occurring during the last 4 weeks of the study period was only 1·5 lb (0·7 kg) compared with an identical mean weight loss of 1·5 lb (0·7 kg) on placebo. Although most studies reveal a similar pattern, it is important to appreciate that there is a wide range of individual weight changes; e.g. in the group of patients studied by Bolding, the individual weight changes occurring on diethylpropion ranged from 0 to a loss of 36 lb, while the weight change of subjects taking placebo varied from a gain of 5 lb to a loss of 22 lb. Likewise, in another 12-week double-blind study, mean weight loss on active drug was 14·9 lb (6·8 kg) and on placebo 9·7 lb (4·4 kg) but the

Table 1 Showing the weight-reducing effect of diethylpropion and placebo given for 12 weeks in the double-blind mode

Authors	Treatment	Total no. of patients	Percentage completing study	Total weight loss (lb (kg))	Weight loss in each 4-week period: (lb (kg))		
					1–4	5–8	9–12
Allen, G. S. (1977)[5]	Drug	40	83	17·5 (7·8)	10·3 (4·7)	4·5 (2·0)	2·7 (1·2)
	Placebo	40	83	10·7 (4·9)	6·2 (2·8)	2·1 (1·0)	2·4 (1·1)
McQuarrie, H. G. D. (1975)[6]	Drug	29	76	9·7 (4·4)	5·1 (2·3)	3·0 (1·4)	1·6 (0·7)
	Placebo	29	66	3·4 (1·5)	0·9 (0·4)	1·3 (0·6)	1·2 (0·5)
Bolding, O. T. (1974)[7]	Drug	25	92	14·8 (6·7)	10·3 (6·7)	4·2 (1·9)	0·0 (0·0)
	Placebo	25	84	9·0 (4·1)	7·0 (3·2)	2·4 (1·1)	0·4 (0·2)
TOTALS	Drug	94	83	14·5 (6·4)	8·3 (3·8)	3·8 (1·7)	1·5 (0·7)
	Placebo	94	78	8·3 (3·8)	4·8 (2·2)	1·9 (0·9)	1·5 (0·7)

individual changes on diethylpropion extended from −6 lb (−2·7 kg) to −33 lb (−15 kg) and on placebo from +23 lb (+10·5 kg) to −24 lb (−10·9 kg)[8].

Patients with hypertensive disease have been successfully treated with diethylpropion without apparent harm. The drug has also been used to control further weight gain occurring in the obese during pregnancy. Although no adverse effects were noted in the babies, in general principles, one is very reluctant to recommend the use of any drug during pregnancy because of uncertainty about teratogenicity. Diethylpropion has also been evaluated in the management of the obesity of childhood and adolescence. It appears to be well tolerated, but generally speaking weight loss is disappointing and there is no evidence to suggest that the weight reduction achieved is of lasting benefit[9].

Doses and availability

Diethylpropion is marketed in the United Kingdom as 25 mg tablets. The recommended dose is one tablet for children over the age of six and three tablets taken 1 h before meals for adolescents and adults. 75 mg tablets of diethylpropion are also available in a sustained release form combined with a special hydrophilic matrix. This permits a one-daily regime at the expense of flexibility in individual dosage. B-complex vitamins have been added to another delayed-release diethylpropion preparation presumably to prevent vitamin deficiency occurring during inappropriate dietary restriction.

Phentermine

Clinical pharmacology

Phentermine hydrochloride is another amphetamine analogue with only weak sympathomimetic and stimulant effects but with marked anorectic properties. Given in a dose of either 15 or 30 mg it will produce a depression of subjective hunger rating comparable to that achieved with therapeutic doses of amphetamine. The anorectic action persists for at least 10 h following its administration as an iron exchange resin complex. In this form, the drug is readily and evenly absorbed, reaching therapeutic levels within an hour and maximal blood concentration after several hours. The drug is largely excreted unchanged in the urine, the rate of renal handling being influenced by the degree of acidity.

Side-effects and contra-indications

No specific cardiovascular studies of phentermine have been performed but various clinical studies have not detected significant changes apart from blood pressure. The side-effects encountered are very similar to those of diethylpropion and include a dry mouth, increased irritability, mild hyperactivity and insomnia. Following a single-dose ingestion of 240 mg a 26-year-old schizophrenic was acutely disturbed, the effect lasting for 2 weeks. There is also one reported case of toxic psychosis attributed to long-term phentermine abuse in a previous amphetamine addict. One case of congenital cataracts has been associated with the administration. It follows that the potential dangers and contra-indications of phentermine and diethylpropion are comparable.

Efficacy

Controlled clinical trials have confirmed that phentermine is an effective anti-obesity agent with a low incidence of side-effects. It has been suggested that the weight-reducing effect of phentermine may continue somewhat longer than that of comparable drugs. In a study which compared 30 mg of phentermine against placebo for a treatment period of 36 weeks a mean weight loss was achieved on drug therapy for 6 months[10]. Likewise a mean weight loss has been observed in a group of diabetics throughout a 6-month period of treatment. However, the total mean weight loss achieved on active therapy was only 11·6 lb (5·3 kg) compared with a mean weight loss of 3·2 lb (1·5 kg) on placebo[11]. Various other studies lasting 14 or 16 weeks have shown mean weight losses to occur throughout the trial periods, but in each study the magnitude of weight change has diminished progressively[12-14]. Thus if the results of these studies are considered together, mean weight change achieved during the 16 weeks of active therapy was 19·9 lb (9·0 kg) and 11·6 lb (5·3 kg) on placebo treatment. The mean weight reduction occurring in each 4-week period was 8·1 lb (3·7 kg), 5·5 lb (2·5 kg), 3·3 lb (1·6 kg) and 2·9 lb (1·3 kg) on active therapy. The respective figures on placebo treatment were 5·7 lb (2·6 kg), 2·7 lb (1·2 kg), 1·7 lb (0·8 kg) and 1·5 lb (0·7 kg). Thus, during the ninth to the twelfth week of therapy, the extra mean weight loss achieved by the drug-treated group was 0·2 kg per week, and between the thirteenth and sixteenth weeks, it was 0·1 kg per week. Although these results compare favourably with those of diethylpropion and mazindol, it would be unwise to draw any firm conclusion because of the paucity of studies of comparable duration with other drugs. Certainly, on the evidence available, it would be presumptuous to suggest that phentermine is significantly more efficacious than the alternative preparations.

Availability

Phentermine is available as a 15 mg and 30 mg sustained-release resin complex. The recommended dose is one tablet daily at breakfast.

Mazindol

Clinical pharmacology

The discovery of mazindol in 1966 made available to the physician an anti-obesity drug with a unique chemical structure but with appetite-suppressant effects comparable to those of amphetamine. In the previous chapter it has been shown that, in spite of its structural dissimilarity, mazindol has a neuropharmacological effect broadly similar to that of amphetamine itself.

The pharmacokinetics of mazindol have been studied in man. However, the methods used to evaluate the absorption, distribution and excretion of the drug cannot distinguish between mazindol and its major metabolites.

The effect of mazindol on carbohydrate and insulin metabolism is controversial. It has been claimed that it could be of particular value in the management of the obese diabetic because its administration is associated with fasting hyperinsulinaemia. Other studies have failed to confirm this finding, and the changes which occur following chronic administration of mazindol in both non-diabetic and diabetic subjects could be consistent with the effects of weight loss alone. However, the acute single-dose administration of mazindol may improve oral glucose tolerance without affecting intravenous glucose tolerance. This suggests that the drug may impair or delay the absorption of glucose from the alimentary tract[15].

Side-effects

Various side-effects have been attributed to mazindol. These are often mild and relatively transient but they may necessitate discontinuing treatment in at least 10% of subjects. The side-effects include not only nervousness, irritability and insomnia but also drowsiness, lethargy and weakness with dizziness. Dry mouth, nausea, constipation, chills and goose flesh may occur, and loss of libido has been reported in a number of studies. More alarming side-effects which have been reported include severe angioneurotic oedema, vomiting with peripheral oedema[16] and violent tremors in a patient taking methyldopa and flurazepam[17]. It has been claimed that mazindol is significantly more likely to cause troublesome side-effects than diethylpropion[18], but this study was not double-blind and could have been influenced by observer bias.

Drug interactions and contraindications

Because mazindol may potentiate the pressor effects of catecholamines, it should not be given in conjunction with sympathomimetic drugs or with antihypertensive agents of the adrenergic neurone block type such as guanethidine and debrisoquine. It has been given in combination with other hypotensive drugs without affecting the blood pressure. It is contra-indicated in severely agitated states, should be avoided during pregnancy and in patients with glaucoma or peptic ulceration.

Given in therapeutic doses, mazindol does not appear to have a sig-nificantly adverse effect on cardiovascular function. Indeed it has been suggested that it is effective and safe when given to patients with stable cardiac disease. In a small double-blind study of such patients, one of the placebo group experienced a worsening of angina. Of the fifteen patients receiving active therapy, two developed atrial fibrillation, one worsening of angina with blackouts and another developed ECG changes[19]. It would therefore be unwise to prescribe mazindol in patients with significant cardiac disease. There are no reported incidences of addiction to mazindol. Non-fatal accidental poisoning has occurred in a 4-year-old child who took 20 mg of mazindol and recovery after 60 mg has occurred.

Efficacy

Numerous clinical studies have demonstrated that mazindol has an effect on 'hunger' rating. It produces significant weight loss when compared double-blind with placebo. Table 2 summarizes the results of twelve such studies undertaken for 12 weeks[16,17,19-28]. Mean weight losses range from 18·9 lb (8·5 kg) to 3·1 lb (1·4 kg) in a study in which mean weight regain occurred after 6 weeks of active therapy[24]. The mean weight loss for all subjects was 14·1 lb (6·8 kg) on the active drug and 8·1 lb (3·7 kg) on placebo, a difference of 0·5 lb (0·23 kg) per week. In one study the rate of weight loss was maintained throughout the trial[21]. In general, however, most weight loss occurred in the first few weeks. Excluding the small study by Bradley[19] in which the data were not presented, the overall mean weight loss achieved in the first 4 weeks of treatment with mazindol was 7·9 lb (3·6 kg) compared with a mean weight loss of only 2·5 lb (1·1 kg) in the last 4 weeks of these studies. This is in keeping with the observation of Conte[29] who, in a 16-week study, found a mean weight loss of 11·4 lb (5·2 kg) in the first 12 weeks but only an additional weight loss of 1·5 lb (0·68 kg) in the following 4 weeks. Generally speaking, there is no firm evidence to suggest that mazindol's biochemical novelty confers on it any important clinical advantages over the other available anorectic agents.

Availability

Mazindol has usually been evaluated on a daily dosage regime of either 2 or 3 mg. The drug is marketed in the United Kingdom as a 2 mg tablet and the recommended dose is one tablet after breakfast.

Table 2 Summary of 12 double-blind direct comparison studies between mazindol and placebo

Authors	No. of patients	Percentage completing Study	Dosage (mg)	Weight loss (lb (kg))		Additional weight loss (kg/wk)	Comments
				Drug	Placebo		
Wallace, A. G.[16]	50	88	2	12·1 (5·5)	5·1 (2·3)	0·26	Hospital clinic
Mackay and Wallace[17]	414	70·5	2	15·8 (7·2)	10·1 (4·5)	0·22	Multi-active GP study
Bradley et al.[19]	39	72	3	9·8 (4·4)	3·8 (1·7)	0·22	Patients with 'stable' cardiac disease
Bandisole and Boshell[20]	64	67	2	11·0 (5·0)	8·0 (3·6)	0·11	Obese diabetics
Schwartz, L. N.[21]	60	100	2	18·5 (8·4)	2·4 (1·1)	0·60	See text
Heber, K. R.[22]	50	80	2	15·2 (6·9)	3·6 (1·6)	0·44	Single practice GP study
Gomez, G.[23]	72	72	2	13·0 (5·9)	5·3 (2·4)	0·29	GP study
Smith et al.[24]	50	84	2	3·1 (1·4)	0·7 (0·3)	0·09	'Refractory obesity' Mean weight regain after 6 weeks
Sharma et al.[25]	116	80	2	1·89 (0·6)	11·8 (5·3)	0·23	Adolescents at 11–18
Allen, G. S.[26]	80	75	3	17·8 (8·1)	10·7 (5·0)	0·25	
Smith, D. E.[27]	90	78	3	9·7 (4·4)	4·9 (2·2)	0·18	Hospital clinic
Sedgwick, J. P.[28]	60	85	2	18·7 (8·5)	14·4 (6·5)	0·17	Single GP practice study
TOTALS	1145	76	2·3	14·1 (6·4)	8·1 (3·7)	0·23	

DRUGS ACTING ON THE SEROTONERGIC SYSTEMS

Fenfluramine
Fenfluramine is currently the only available drug thought to act primarily on the serotonergic system.

Clinical pharmacology
The absorption, metabolism and excretion of fenfluramine has been extensively studied[30]. The drug is usually absorbed rapidly and virtually completely from the alimentary tract. Following a single dose, maximum plateau concentrations are achieved after 2–4 h. Fenfluramine is widely distributed throughout the body, accumulating in the liver, brain, kidney, heart and to a lesser extent in muscle and adipose tissue. It is rapidly metabolized into the de-ethylated active derivative norfenfluramine. Both fenfluramine and norfenfluramine are excreted in the urine, the rate of excretion being very dependent upon urinary pH, rising when the urine is acidic. Possibly because of tissue storage and protein binding, the mean plasma half-life of fenfluramine, and also of norfenfluramine, is about 20 h. On a fixed daily dose regime, plasma concentrations will build up to reach a plateau state after 3–4 days. However, pharmacokinetic studies in healthy volunteers or in patients have shown that there are very considerable variations in the steady-state concentrations reached when using a fixed dosage regime. It has also been shown that plasma concentrations correlate closely with the degree of subjective appetite suppression[30].

Side-effects
Some patients can tolerate large doses of fenfluramine without experiencing troublesome side-effects. A few cannot take small quantities without becoming unwell and may complain of drowsiness, depression, lethargy or even a sensation of unreality. Although there are isolated instances when this sensation of de-personalization resulted in drug abuse, generally speaking, fenfluramine has the great clinical advantage of not causing CNS stimulation. However, fenfluramine does alter cerebral function during sleep in a manner similar to that of the stimulant amphetamines. There are alterations in EEG slow wave sleep, dose-related reductions in para-doxical sleep and increase in intra-sleep restlessness. This latter probably accounts for the reported increase in dreaming and nightmares. Dreaming may be dose-related but is especially liable to become clinically apparent when the dose is being increased or reduced. Abrupt discontinuation of treatment causes rebound abnormalities of sleep. These changes are maxi-mal after 3–4 days, in keeping with the pharmacokinetics of the drug and also with the timing of post-withdrawal depression. This can be very severe and is probably fenfluramine's greatest disadvantage. Its occurrence

can, however, be minimized if the drug is discontinued slowly and stepwise.

Gastrointestinal side-effects of fenfluramine include a dry mouth with thirst and sometimes a metallic taste. Nausea, vomiting and colicky abdominal pains have been infrequently reported, but diarrhoea is relatively common, affecting over 10% of all patients. It sometimes is very troublesome though it tends to wear off if treatment can be continued. Other possible side-effects include an increased susceptibility to convulsions in epileptics, urinary frequency, changes in libido and alopecia, though it is uncertain if any or all of these are causally related.

Generally speaking, it would appear that the instance of side-effects is dose-related but can be reduced if patients are started on a low dose which is then increased stepwise over a period of several weeks.

Drug interactions and contraindications
Fenfluramine affects the activity of a number of psychotrophic drugs, and may potentiate the anti-depressant effect of the tricyclic drugs. Because of the potential risk of withdrawal depression, fenfluramine is best avoided in patients requiring any anxiolytic agent. It should not be given in conjunction with a monoamine oxidase inhibitor because this combination has produced acute confusion. The drug is also contraindicated during the first trimester of pregnancy and in epileptics.

Fenfluramine may have a blood pressure lowering effect, expecially when given in conjunction with hypertensive drugs. This can be a therapeutic advantage in the obese hypertensive but the administration or withdrawal of fenfluramine may necessitate making changes in hypotensive therapy. Likewise, fenfluramine can potentiate the therapeutic efficacy of a conventional oral hypoglycaemic agent, the dose of which may require appropriate adjusting during periods of fenfluramine administration or after its withdrawal.

Over-dosage
Although the drug is relatively non-toxic, excessive over-dosage can be life-threatening. Features of acute over-dosage may include hyperpyrexia, dilated non-reactive pupils, rotatory nystagmus, hyperventilation, tachycardia with nausea, abdominal pain and vomiting. Agitation may progress to dreaming and rarely coma. The treatment is largely symptomatic but a forced acid diuresis will produce considerable increase in urinary excretion. Acute confusion or convulsions may require treatment with diazepam. The patient requires continuous ECG monitoring and anti-arrhythmic drugs may be necessary.

Clinical efficacy
Fenfluramine has been extensively evaluated in a large number of double-

blind, direct-comparison studies which have confirmed that it produces weight loss superior to that obtained by placebo. As with other agents, the maximum weight loss is usually observed during the initial period of therapy, and there is considerable variability in the response of different subjects. It has been suggested that high doses of fenfluramine are no more effective than those conventionally prescribed. However, in a recent 20-week study in female patients with refractory obesity, there was a direct relationship between plasma fenfluramine and norfenfluramine concentrations and weight loss; subjects whose mean fenfluramine concentration was less than 100 ng/ml only achieving a mean weight loss of 4·6 lb (2·1 kg) while those with levels between 100 and 199 ng/ml, and those in excess of 200 ng/ml, achieved mean weight losses of 11·2 lb (5·1 kg) and 19·4 lb (8·8 kg) respectively[31] (see Figure 1). There was no significant difference in the mean stated dose of fenfluramine and either the weight loss or the plasma drug concentrations. Failure to achieve therapeutically

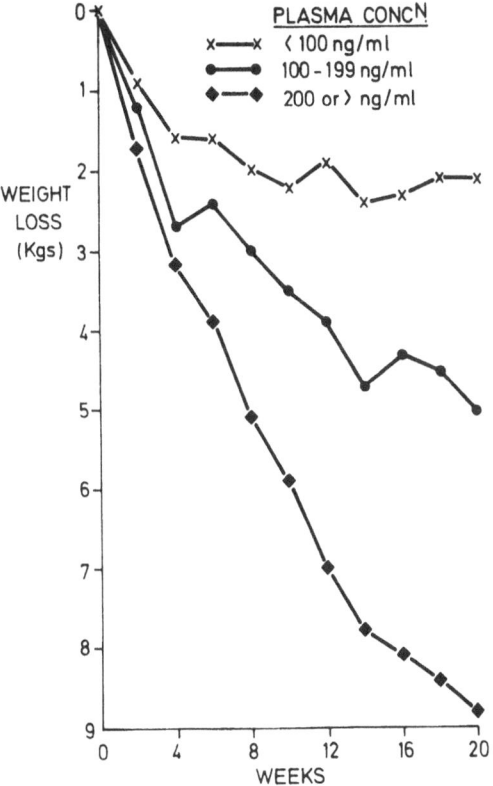

Figure 1 The relationship between mean plasma fenfluramine concentrations and mean weight loss achieved in female subjects with refractory obesity during a 20-week study (from *Br. Med. J.* by permission of the editor)

effective concentrations can sometimes be attributed to the prior development of troublesome side-effects, but in others must be due either to poor patient compliance or to individual differences either in drug absorption or metabolism. Further experience has shown that some subjects will fail to lose weight even with plasma fenfluramine concentrations in excess of 200 ng/ml, but generally speaking, when fenfluramine is prescribed the dose should be increased stepwise either until satisfactory weight loss occurs or until troublesome side-effects develop. Because of its possible hypotensive and mild hypoglycaemic properties, fenfluramine may be of additional value in the management of obesity complicated by hypertension or diabetes. Certainly, it has now been shown that the blood glucose-lowering effect is greater than that which can be attributed to weight loss alone[32].

Availability
Fenfluramine is marketed as a 20 mg tablet and as a 60 mg sustained-release capsule. There is no evidence that the capsule is therapeutically more effective. Although it could be argued that the use of the capsule may improve patient compliance, it also restricts the ability to titrate the dose of drug to the individual's requirements.

OTHER DRUGS

The previous chapter has emphasized the variety of ways whereby pharmacological agents may produce weight loss. One such drug is hydroxycitrate, which has yet to be evaluated in man. The use of dietary fibre has been discussed in the chapter on diets. Various other agents however are, or in the past have been, used for their anti-obesity effect. They include the following:

Biguanides

Clinical pharmacology
The biguanides have been used in the management of insulin-independent diabetics for 20 years. They lower the blood glucose in the diabetic but not in the non-diabetic except in severe over-dosage. They do not stimulate insulin release, and their exact mode of action is still uncertain. They delay gastric emptying, inhibit the absorption of glucose, amino acids and other nutrients from the alimentary tract, and enhance glycolysis and decrease glucogenesis from alanine pyruvate and lactate. This results in an increase in blood lactate and a susceptibility to lactic acidosis. Phenformin is partly metabolized in the liver and partly excreted unchanged in the urine,

whereas metformin is totally excreted by the kidneys. It follows that the plasma concentration and half-life of both drugs is increased in the presence of renal impairment, but hepatic dysfunction only affects phenformin.

Side-effects
Phenformin and metformin are reasonably well tolerated but can cause gastrointestinal upsets. These include anorexia, nausea, a metallic taste, diarrhoea and, less frequently, abdominal pain and vomiting. These side-effects can be minimized by giving a small initial dose and gradually increasing the drug which should be taken in divided doses with meals. Prolonged administration may result in sub-clinical malabsorption of B_{12}.

The most important side-effects of the biguanides is the risk of lactic acidosis which has proved fatal in about half the reported cases. Usually, there is an underlying associated condition, especially renal, hepatic or cardiac insufficiency. Occasionally lactic acidosis can arise without explanation soon after initiating treatment with, or increasing the dosage of, phenformin. Lactic acidosis is much less likely to occur with metformin, possibly because phenformin may more adversely affect the clearance of a lactate load. Metformin-induced lactic acidosis is almost invariably associated with renal failure.

Drug interactions and contraindications
The biguanides should be used only with great caution if there is any degree of renal insufficiency, and are contraindicated in patients with renal failure. The risk of lactic acidosis can be minimized by avoiding treatment if the serum creatinine is greater than 1·2 mg/dl. Biguanides should not be prescribed if there is any other chronic condition which may cause lactic acidosis, such as cardiac or hepatic insufficiency or alcoholism. They must also be withdrawn in the event of an acute intercurrent illness such as myocardial infarction or fulminating infection, which may precipitate hypotensive shock and lead to tissue hypoxia.

Because of the fibrinolytic effects of the biguanides special care must also be taken during concomitant anticoagulation administration.

Efficacy
The weight-reducing properties of the biguanides are probably multifactorial. They may be partly due to a reduction in food intake caused by anorexia, but reduction in food consumption alone does not account for all the weight loss achieved in the diabetic or obese non-diabetic[33]. Possibly the biguanides diminish absorption of nutrients from the alimentary tract, or possibly they have a more fundamental effect on carbohydrate or lipid metabolism.

The Diabetic – Although the University Group Diabetes Programme Report drew attention to the potential hazards of oral hypoglycaemic therapy, such drugs are still widely prescribed. There is general agreement that the addition of a biguanide may result in weight loss or at least prevent weight gain in the obese diabetic in spite of achieving an improvement in diabetic control. Metformin and phenformin are equally effective[34]. The rate of weight loss is less marked in subjects also receiving sulphonylurea[35], in contrast with weight gain in patients whose glycosuria is controlled by sulphonylurea alone[36]. Weight loss is most marked during the first few months of treatment, and mean weight loss may cease after 6–12 months of therapy[36,37]. In a retrospective analysis of 168 diabetics treated with a biguanide for at least 5 years, there was a mean weight loss of 13 lb (6 kg) and only 9% of the patients gained weight[38]. Some studies failed to relate weight loss to dosage regime, but in others a greater reduction has occurred in patients receiving a higher dosage. It has been suggested that weight reduction is less likely to occur in the least over-weight[39]. However, two prospective cross-over studies in obese and non-obese diabetics have compared the weight change achieved during 12 months of treatment with metformin to that obtained during a year's therapy with chlorpropamide. In obese diabetics the difference was 14·3 lb (6·5 kg)[36] while in the non-obese diabetic, the difference was almost identical at 13·4 lb (6·1 kg)[40]. In both instances, the major change was due to weight gain while receiving the sulphonylurea. It would be attractive to suggest that if the biguanides' weight-reducing properties are not primarily due to their anorectic effect, then the addition of a conventional 'appetite-suppressant' might enhance their effect. Unfortunately, the available evidence does not substantiate this possibility[11]. Nonetheless, increasing obesity in an already overweight and poorly controlled diabetic is clearly undesirable. In such patients, an effective treatment is metformin.

The non-diabetic – The various studies have shown no significant weight loss in non-diabetics, and it has been suggested that the biguanides will only produce weight reduction in subjects who are diabetic or who have a family history of diabetes[37,41]. Possibly, in view of the complexity of the metabolic changes that are associated with obesity and diabetes it may be inappropriate to make an arbitrary distinction between the obese diabetic and the non-diabetic on the grounds of an oral glucose tolerance test. Certainly, other studies have demonstrated substantial weight loss in non-diabetic adults[33,42,43], and children[44]. It is possible that the non-diabetic will only lose weight if the dosage is increased up to, but not beyond, that required to produce side-effects. Even then, however, the weight loss is less than that obtained with fenfluramine[43]. The biguanides have not been directly compared with other anorectic agents. At high doses, the risk of lactic acidosis is increased and further long-term studies will have to be undertaken before the biguanides can be recommended in the management of the obese non-diabetic. Possibly they may prove to be of value not so much in promoting weight loss as in preventing weight gain following effective dietary treatment.

Thyroid hormones

Introduction

The basal metabolic rate (BMR) or non-shivering thermogenesis usually accounts for about half of the total daily energy requirements. Since thyroid hormones greatly modify the BMR, the influence of thyroid function in the aetiology of obesity and the therapeutic potential of thyroid hormones in its management have been extensively evaluated. Generally speaking, thyroid function tests, including T_3 suppression of radio-iodine thyroid gland uptake, are normal in obesity. However, it is possible that obesity may be associated with an increased peripheral resistance to thyroid hormones. There is also increasing evidence that an alteration in carbohydrate intake, with or without overall change in energy consumption, will produce an alteration in the proportion of thyroxine (T_4) converted into tri-iodothyronine (T_3) or into its physiologically inert isomer (reverse T_3 or RT_3). The ratio of T_3 to RT_3 normally increases during overfeeding with carbohydrates and falls when dietary carbohydrate is reduced. This reduction in the ratio of T_3 to RT_3 may either reflect, or indeed be an integral part of, an adaptive process to dietary restriction. It seems possible that changes in this physiological control mechanism may explain why some subjects appear to gain weight so easily and why others fail to lose weight in spite of an appropriate reduction in energy intake[45]. If this were the case, such subjects might be expected to respond to treatment with thyroid hormones.

Clinical pharmacology

Both T_3 and T_4 are well absorbed from the small intestine. Approximately 40% of T_4 is converted in the liver to T_3 and subsequently excreted in the biliary and renal tract. Circulating T_4 is almost completely protein-bound but T_3 is less protein-bound and the biological potency of T_3 is four to five times greater than T_4, and 10 μg of T_3 are approximately equivalent to 50 μg of T_4. The plasma half-lives of T_3 and T_4 are 2 days and 7 days respectively.

Mode of action

Thyroid hormones are believed to increase the activity of the membrane-bound enzyme ATP which controls the intracellular/extracellular sodium and potassium gradients. In addition, they may increase the activity of the mitochondrial enzyme glycerophosphate dehydrogenase, which oxidizes glycerol-3 phosphate and so diverts glycerol from the pathway of triglyceride synthesis. T_3 may also influence protein synthesis by facilitating the transcription of DNA.

Much of the weight loss during thyroid hormone therapy is due to a reduction of lean body mass, fat loss being only minimally affected. There is a marked increase in nitrogen loss maximal within the first 10 days of treatment but persisting for at least 1 month and probably longer. Protein losses, however, can be prevented either by increasing the dietary intake of protein or by the use of anabolic steroids and growth hormone.

Drug interactions and toxicity

Common symptoms of T_3 and T_4 toxicity include nervousness, excessive sweating, palpitations, tiredness and an increase in bowel frequency. The thyroid hormones should be used with great caution in patients with cardiovascular disease, as they may produce systolic hypertension and aggravate angina. Indeed, a potential, serious, long-term side-effect is the development of thyrotoxic cardiomyopathy.

The thyroid hormones enhance the effects of digoxin, oral anticoagulants and tricyclic antidepressants. In addition, the effect of the thyroid hormones may be increased by phenytoin, tricyclic antidepressants and aspirin. These interactions are probably due to drug displacement from the serum proteins. Thyroid hormones may also antagonize the action of various drugs used in the control of diabetes mellitus and in susceptible individuals are diabetogenic.

Efficacy in obesity

Various studies have shown that pharmacological doses of thyroid abstract are remarkably well tolerated by the obese, and when combined with dietary restriction, enhance weight loss in some patients[46,47]. In a double-blind 12-week study the addition of physiological doses of thyroid hormone (thyroid extract 180 mg daily) significantly enhanced and prolonged the weight loss of patients treated with dexamphetamine but without dietary restriction[48]. The 53 patients completing the study who received dexamphetamine alone, achieved a mean weight loss of 0·94 lb (0·42 kg) per week, differing significantly from the 48 patients receiving the combination, whose mean weight loss was 1·2 lb (0·55 kg) per week. However, in both groups, weight loss had plateaued at 10 weeks.

In another study in which patients were either given T_3 or T_4, the dose was increased stepwise to the maximum tolerated, resulting in a mean dose of T_3 of 275 μg per day and a mean dose of T_4 of 1·4 mg per day. Four of the 17 patients failed to complete the study, two because of intolerable nervousness and tachycardia and two because of the development of glycosuria with hyperglycaemia. A placebo group gained weight while the treated patients lost on average 0·95 lb (0·44 kg) each week. There was no significant difference observed in the weight loss achieved between the two treatment groups, and surprisingly no evidence of tolerance developed even after 30 weeks. However, following the cessation of thyroid hormone therapy, weight regain recurred rapidly. Others have confirmed the efficacy of T_3 versus the placebo using 225 μg of T_3 daily in thirteen massively obese subjects on an 800-calorie diet[49]. Clearly, however, the indiscriminate use of thyroid hormones in the management of obesity uncomplicated by hypothyroidism cannot be justified. Their use may be indicated in a small, clearly defined sub-group in whom metabolic studies have shown a severe reduction of energy consumption. Even then, however, their use should be restricted to the relatively young patient free from cardiovascular, renal or hepatic disease. A supplemented protein intake should be given to avoid negative nitrogen balance. The drugs should be prescribed to the maximum tolerated dose and continued for longer than is customary when using anorectic agents. There are good reasons for suggesting that T_3 may be a more appropriate form of treatment than either thyroid extract or T_4. However, in view of the long-term risks, further long-term studies are required to evaluate these drugs before their use can be recommended.

Human chorionic gonadotrophins
The rationale behind the use of gonadotrophin is uncertain. Although the evidence is conflicting, it is probably ineffective[50,51].

Cholestyramine
The success of intestinal bypass surgery has provided a stimulus to examine the possibility of producing drug-induced malabsorption. Cholestyramine reduces fat absorption by binding bile acids, and is used to control the chemical diarrhoea caused by unbound bile acids in the large bowel. Although it will increase faecal fat excretion, the dosage required to produce a worthwhile change is clinically unacceptable and subjects discontinue treatment[52].

Bromocriptine
Bromocriptine specifically reduces prolactin secretion and is effective in supressing purpural lactation. It has various other therapeutic indications and substantial weight loss has occurred during prolonged treatment[53]. Although bromocriptine normally raises growth hormone levels in the non-obese, it does not correct the abnormally low plasma growth hormone

concentrations of morbid obesity nor does it produce any consistent change in weight when given to such subjects for 3 months at a dose of 10 mg per day[54]. Its use as an anti-obesity agent cannot be justified.

Levo-dopa

Because of its gastrointestinal side-effects, which include nausea and vomiting, levo-dopa has been evaluated in a double-blind study[55]. However, it is not an effective weight-reducing agent and indeed has been used in the management of anorexia nervosa[56]!

THE CHOICE OF DRUG

Opinions regarding the value of drug therapy in obesity vary widely. Some believe that drugs are a valuable adjunct to conventional therapy while others feel that they are ineffective and potentially dangerous. Clinical comparison of different anti-obesity agents is bedevilled by the problems discussed in the previous chapter. At present, the only reliable index for comparison is that of weight loss. This fails to take into consideration the therapeutic significance of such factors as possible differences in the mode of action of the various drugs.

The FDA Report

The Food and Drug Administration have recently analysed the results of more than 200 short-term studies involving almost 10 000 patients. Only trials designed in the double-blind mode, with a control group receiving either placebo or another appetite-suppressant drug, were included in the analysis. Various active preparations included amphetamine, metamphetamine, phenmetrazine, benzphetamine, phentermine, chlorphentermine, diethylpropion, mazindol and fenfluramine. Computer analysis of the results showed that almost half of all the subjects undergoing treatment did not complete these short-duration trials. The dropout rates were comparable between placebo and active groups. These high default rates influence the interpretation of the data. However, in over 90% of the studies, the active drug produced a greater weight loss than placebo, though the additional weight lost was neither great nor invariable, the difference between active and placebo groups being only statistically significant in 40% of the studies. The pooled results of the analysis are shown in Table 3[57]. After 4 weeks of treatment, subjects taking an active drug, lost on average 0·56 lb (0·25 kg) per week more than those taking the placebo. Irrespective of the duration of the individual studies, the overall additional weight loss attributable to drug treatment was approximately 0·5 lb (0·23 kg) per week.

Table 3 Summary of analysis of FDA review of clinical trials comparing weight loss on placebo or active drug

	Placebo	*Active drug*
Number of patients	4543	3182
Dropouts (percentage)		
4 weeks of treatment	18·5	24·5
End of study	49·0	47·9
Weight loss achieved (percentage)		
1 lb per week	26	44
3 lb per week	1	2
Weight loss achieved over 4 weeks (percentage)		
1 lb per week	46	68
3 lb per week	4	10

By permission of Professor G. A. Bray, Editor of *Obesity and Perspective*, and Dr B. A. Scoville.

In their final report, the working party emphasized that whereas the natural history of obesity is measured in years, the studies they had analysed were restricted to a few weeks' duration. They felt that the total impact of drug-induced weight loss must be considered to be clinically trivial. Although the amount of weight loss varied from one study to another, they were unable to discriminate between one drug and another, and felt that variability in weight loss related to factors other than the drug prescribed, such as dietary advice and patient selection.

Studies in refractory obesity

One way of overcoming the problem of variability in patient selection is to study subjects in whom the weight problem has become intractable. Such patients have been investigated in Edinburgh, where subjects are defined as having refractory obesity if they fulfil the following criteria:

1. female subjects;
2. have previously attended a special hospital clinic for not less than 12 months;
3. have been advised to take a diet based on the principle of carbohydrate restriction and designed to provide 1000 kcal (4·18 MJ) per day;
4. have failed to lose weight during the 3 months preceding the study;
5. have now received an anti-obesity agent for at least 3 months;
6. are not clinically oedematous

Figure 2 shows the mean weight losses achieved in a series of separate double-blind studies during which a variety of anti-obesity drugs were administered for 12 weeks to subjects who fulfilled these criteria of

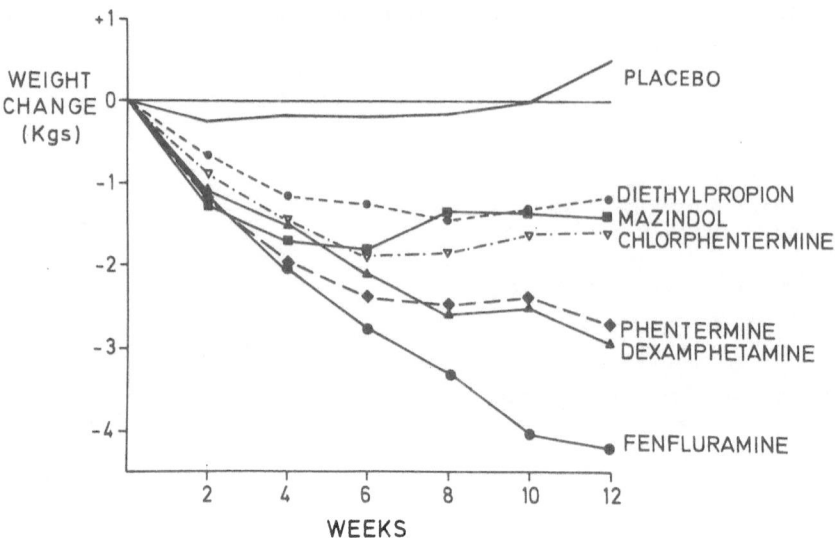

Figure 2 Weight loss achieved by placebo and various anti-obesity agents in female patients with refractory obesity (by permission of the Symposium Editor of the Royal College of Physicians, Edinburgh)

refractory obesity[24,58,61]. The differences and similarities between the groups of patients studies are shown in Table 4. In these studies the overall dropout rate was 13% on placebo therapy and 14% on active treatment. The validity of the definition of refractory obesity is reflected by the fact that the mean change in subjects receiving placebo therapy was +0·03 lb (0·01 kg) per week. Although the mean weight losses achieved by the anti-obesity drugs ranged from 2·5 lb (1.1 kg) on diethylpropion to 9·3 lb (4·2 kg) on fenfluramine, the figure emphasizes the similarity in the mean weight losses, rather than the differences. The overall mean weight loss that occurred on active therapy was 5·1 lb (2·3 kg) or 0·43 lb (0·19 kg) per week. However, the mean weight loss in the first 4 weeks was 3·6 lb (1·6 kg) and in the last 4 weeks only 0·3 lb (0·13 kg). This would imply, if nothing else, that when given in a fixed dosage regime, the weight-reducing effect of these anti-obesity drugs (with the possible exception of fenfluramine) diminishes during continuous administration for periods of up to 12 weeks in most subjects with refractory obesity. However, a small number of patients achieved impressive individual weight loss and thus maximum weight losses achieved for each of the drugs were diethylpropion 10 lb (4·5 kg)[58]; chlorphentermine 14 lb (6·4 kg)[60]; dexamphetamine 15 lb (6·8 kg)[59]; phentermine 15 lb (6·8 kg)[59]; mazindol 19 lb (8·6 kg)[24]; and fenfluramine 20 lb (9·1 kg)[61]. Thus, the individual variability in response to an anti-obesity agent persists even among patients with refractory obesity. Indeed, these studies in refractory obesity would

Table 4 Showing differences and similarities between groups of patients with refractory obesity studied with various appetite-suppressive agents

Drug	Daily dosage regime (mg)	Number of patients	Mean age (years)	Mean percentage in excess of ideal weight	Percentage completing study
Placebo	—	100	51	44·1	87
Diethylpropion	100	24	54	41·7	83
Mazindol	2	25	47	53	78
Chlorphentermine	75	21	57	44	95
Phentermine	30	23	57	43	100
Dexamphetamine	15	23	58	41	83
Fenfluramine	80	30	49	44·7	83

merely appear to confirm the conclusions of the FDA working party that the major variability is the individual's response to drug treatment, rather than the efficacy of one drug compared with another.

Double-blind comparative studies

A number of double-blind studies have contrasted the efficacy of one drug with another, either by direct comparison or by using the cross-over technique. Three cross-over studies have contrasted fenfluramine with diethylpropion[62-64]. Twice, each drug was given for 4 weeks, and in the third study each drug was prescribed for 8 weeks. The mean weight losses achieved per week on fenfluramine were 1·44 lb (0·65 kg), 0·68 lb (0·31 kg) and 0·45 lb (0·20 kg), the corresponding losses for diethylpropion being 1·36 lb (0·62 kg), 1·1 lb (0·5 kg) and 0·41 lb (0·19 kg). None of the differences is statistically significant. In a further cross-over study, 8 weeks therapy with fenfluramine produced a weekly mean weight loss of 1·43 lb (0·69 kg) which was significantly greater than that achieved using metformin 1·5 g per day (0·99 lb or 0·45 kg per week) and using metformin 3·5 g per day where the weight losses achieved were even less[43].

The results of six double-blind direct-comparison studies lasting for 6 weeks or more have been summarized in Table 5[23,26,65-68]. The drugs evaluated were D-amphetamine, mazindol, fenfluramine and phentermine. The intermittent treatment regime used in the 36 weeks study comprised 4 weeks of active therapy followed by 4 weeks on matching placebo. The results of the weight changes are presented in terms of mean weight loss per week of therapy. Intermittent fenfluramine was less effective than either continuous fenfluramine or intermittent phentermine[65]. One of the studies comparing mazindol with D-amphetamine[23] found the former to be significantly more effective. In all the other studies, however, the weight losses achieved were remarkably similar and the general impression is that the mean weight-reducing property of one 'appetite-suppressant' is much the same as the other.

Comparison of intermittent and continuous therapy

The intermittent use of fenfluramine is not only relatively ineffective[65] but is also associated with a high incidence of side-effects. It is generally agreed that fenfluramine should therefore be given continuously throughout a course of therapy. This may distinguish fenfluramine from other available drugs. Various studies have evalued the continuous and intermittent use of methylpropion[4,6,8,26,62,63,69], mazindol[29,70] and phentermine[10,31](Table 6). Although most studies involved the alternative administration of 4 weeks active and 4 weeks placebo therapy, other regimes may be as effective. The results show that intermittent therapy can be recommended with these drugs on the grounds that it would appear to be as effective, and

Table 5 Analysis of double-blind direct comparison studies lasting for more than 6 weeks

Authors	Duration (weeks)	No. of patients	Percentage completing study	Drug	Dose (mg/day)	Weight loss per week (lb (kg))	Comment
Stunkard, A. et al.[66]	7	60	52	Fenfluramine D-amphetamine	60–120 15– 30	0·96 (0·42) 0·88 (0·40)	High default rate; results comparable
Allen, G. S.[26]	8	80	74	Diethylpropion Mazindol	75 3	1·85 (0·84) 1·90 (0·90)	A placebo test 0·89 lb (0·4 kg) per week
Vernace, B. J.[67]	12	70	89	Mazindol D-amphetamine	3 15	1·17 (0·53) 1·09 (0·49)	Placebo group lost 0.47 lb (0·21 kg) per week
Gomez, G.[23]	12	90	64	Mazindol Fenfluramine	2 120	1·08 (0·49) 0·90 (0·40)	Placebo group lost 0·58 lb (0·26 kg) per week
Kornhaber, A.[68]	12	28	93	Mazindol D-amphetamine	3 15	1·55 (0·70) 0·82 (0·37)	Significant difference on a small group of subjects
Steel, J. M. et al.[65]	36	105	77	Fenfluramine Intermittent fenfluramine Intermittent phentermine	60 60 30	0·72 (0·32) 0·48 (0·21) 0·73 (0·32)	Intermittent therapy comprising 4 weeks on active drug alternative with 4 weeks on placebo

Table 6 Analysis of studies comparing intermittent and continuous treatment with various anti-obesity agents

Authors	Drug	Daily dose (mg)	Duration (weeks)	Nature of intermittent therapy	Mean weight loss in lb (and kg)		
					Continuous	Intermittent	Placebo
Nolan, G. R.[8]	Diethylpropion	75	12	4 weeks active/4 weeks placebo	14·1(6·4)	13·4(6·1)	9·7(9·4)
McQuarrie, H. G.[6]	Diethylpropion	75	12	4 weeks active/4 weeks placebo	9·7(4·4)	6·6(3·0)	3·4(1·5)
Allen, G. S.[26]	Diethylpropion	75	12	4 weeks active/4 weeks placebo	20·0(9·1)	15·4(7·0)	9·8(4·5)
Silverstone, T.[69]	Diethylpropion	75	16	4 weeks active/4 weeks placebo	18·0(8·2)	14·3(6·5)	—
Conte, A.[29]	Mazindol	3	16	4 weeks active/2 weeks placebo	12·9(5·9)	11·0(5·0)	6·7(3·0)
Asher, W. L.[70]*	Mazindol	3	16	4 weeks active/2 weeks placebo	12·9(5·9)	17·0(7·7)	8·6(3·9)
Truant, A. P. et al.[13]	Phentermine	30	16	3 weeks active/1 week placebo	20·3(9·2)	18·4(8·4)	11·5(5·2)
Le Riche, W. H. and Csima, A.[4]	Diethylpropion	75	24	4 weeks active/4 weeks placebo	14·5(6·6)	25·0(11·4)	—
Munro, J. F. et al.[10]	Phentermine	30	36	4 weeks active/4 weeks placebo	27·0(12·3)	28.7(13·0)	10·5(4·8)

* personal communication

is cheaper and presumably less likely to lead in the long term to drug misuse.

Cost

If the relative efficacy of the available drugs is similar the ultimate choice should depend upon additional considerations such as the inherent risks of therapy and the frequency and severity of the side-effects. These aspects have already been discussed. A further factor which cannot be ignored is cost. The cost of 4 weeks of treatment on conventional dosage regimes of preparations currently available in Britain is shown in Table 7.

Table 7 Relative cost of 1 month's anti-obesity treatment (from *MIMS*, October 1978)

Approved name	*Proprietary name*	*Dosage regime (per day)*	*Cost (£)*
Amphetamine and Dexamphetamine in equal parts	Durophet	12·5 mg	0·97
Phenmetrazine, 30 mg Phenbutrazate, 30 mg	Filon	2 tabs	2·35
Diethylpropion	Apisate	75 mg	0·47
	Tenuate Dospan	75 mg	0·72
	Tenuate	75 mg	0·81
Phentermine	Duromine	30 mg	1·96
	Ionamin	30 mg	1·26
Fenfluramine	Ponderax, tabs	120 mg	6·14
	Ponderax, pacaps	120 mg	6·82
Mazindol	Teronac	2 mg	3·13

CHOICE OF PATIENT

It has been previously emphasized that there is more to the management of obesity than mere weight loss. Indeed, many patients with a weight problem will consult their doctor for some specific reason other than their obesity. It follows that weight reduction must be considered within the concept of an overall management plan. The use of anti-obesity drugs however can only be justified in the context of:

  (i) promoting weight loss;
 (ii) preventing further weight gain;
(iii) preventing weight regain following successful weight reduction.

Until these subjects at high risk of gaining weight can be identified it would be difficult to evaluate or justify the use of anti-obesity drugs in a purely prophylactic role. At present, their value in preventing weight regain after drastic weight reduction brought about by such manoeuvres as inpatient starvation, dental splinting or protein-sparing fasting, has not been assessed. This is unfortunate because of the generally disappointing long-term results of these 'drastic cures'. It follows that at present their clinical use is almost exclusively restricted to their role in promoting weight loss.

It is inappropriate to prescribe an anti-obesity drug if the patient is opposed to its use. It would be equally inappropriate to suggest that they should be given merely because the subject asks for them. Unfortunately, this may be a common reason for their prescription. The individual practitioner may find it easier to acquiesce to a request for slimming tablets than to explore the alternative, and relatively time-consuming, forms of treatment. However, in some subjects an appetite-suppressant drug will bring about dramatic weight loss. Possibly, in the past, too much attention has been devoted to comparing one agent with another and too little attention to contrasting one patient with another. There have been few attempts to explain why some subjects fail to benefit from an anti-obesity agent while others do well.

Drug compliance

One obvious explanation is poor drug compliance. There is mounting evidence that many subjects take prescribed drugs infrequently or not at all. This is particularly the case if:

(i) the drug has to be administered several times a day;
(ii) there is no immediate tangible benefit from treatment;
(iii) treatment is associated with troublesome side-effects.

The incidence of poor drug compliance in the management of obesity is largely anecdotal, but there is no doubt that sometimes failure of drug therapy can be attributed to failure of the subjects to take their medicine.

Metabolic considerations

The causes of 'simple' obesity are complex, remain poorly defined and are almost certainly multifactorial. However, with regard to drug therapy, subjects can be broadly divided into three categories:

(i) Subjects with normal energy expenditure who have gained weight because of excessive food intake but who are capable of altering their dietary habits thereby producing a sufficient 'energy gap' to cause effective weight loss without recourse to appetite-suppressants. Clearly, in such subjects drug therapy is unnecessary.

(ii) Similar subjects who for one reason or another are unable to control their food intake. Some will be aware of their inability to curb their 'appetite' but others may delude themselves into thinking that they are failing to lose weight while adhering to a strict dietary regime. In either case, the administration of an appetite-suppressant could result in dramatic weight loss.

(iii) Subjects who have a low energy expenditure and therefore will fail to lose weight while adhering to a 'slimming regime'[45]. Such subjects, who have already reduced their energy intake, are unlikely to benefit from the administration of a drug which works primarily by curbing the appetite. In them, to be effective, drug therapy would have to increase their metabolic rate rather than reduce their already diminished food intake.

Clearly there is no absolute distinction between one category and another. Indeed it is possible that subjects can 'move' into a different category as a result of metabolic adaptation to a low energy intake. For example, the fact that weight loss plateaus 1–2 years after bypass surgery may in part be due to increased food intake, and partly to physiological changes that occur in the segment of small intestine in continuity but it may also reflect a metabolic adaptation to sustained reduction in energy intake.

Drug tolerance
This concept may be highly relevant when considering the problem of drug tolerance. It is generally considered that the tendency for drug-induced weight loss to diminish with time is an index of the development of 'drug tolerance' and is an indication to discontinue treatment. While not wishing to belittle the importance of drug tolerance, it is possible that sometimes the levelling off in weight loss may reflect metabolic adaptation, or what might be regarded as 'patient tolerance'. This is in keeping with the observations of Enzi and his colleagues[71] who gave mazindol intermittently to a small group of subjects for over a year. They found that although the weight-reducing effect of the regime gradually diminished, the degree of subjective suppression of appetite persisted throughout their lengthy study. If an appetite-suppressant drug produces a significant reduction in food intake, weight loss will occur. After an interval of time, the body may react to the 'energy gap' that has been created by reducing energy expenditure. If this were the case, then the discontinuation of an appetite-suppressant drug would almost certainly be associated with weight regain.

Effects of drug withdrawal on weight
There is considerable evidence that most subjects regain the weight lost during treatment after the drug is withdrawn. For example, after the

completion of a double-blind study which compared mazindol and
D-amphetamine with placebo, there was a mean increase in weight in
patients who had been treated with an active preparation, whereas those
who had received placebo had a further reduction in mean weight. After
$2\frac{1}{2}$ years, the mean weight changes of three groups were comparable[68].
Similarly, although diethylpropion produced substantial weight loss in
children, a follow-up undertaken 1 year later showed no long-term benefit
from the drug therapy[9]. In a single-practice GP study of 176 patients, the
mean weight loss achieved during 12 months treatment with fenfluramine
was 22 lb (10 kg). During the 1-year of follow up period, there was a mean
weight regain of nearly 20 lb (9·1 kg)[71]. Mean change in weight was most
rapid at the onset and after the withdrawal of therapy. Likewise, substantial weight regain has been reported within 6 weeks of discontinuing
treatment with phentermine[12] and other short-term, double-blind, cross-
over studies which have compared various active drugs with placebo, have
all demonstrated that the mean weight loss achieved after drug therapy and
while receiving placebo is very insubstantial[72-74].

Similar studies of longer duration further illustrate the problem. For
example, the mean weight loss obtained during 11 weeks of fenfluramine
increasing to 160 mg per day was more than regained during 11 weeks on
placebo therapy[43] (see Figure 3). Likewise, the weight loss achieved by

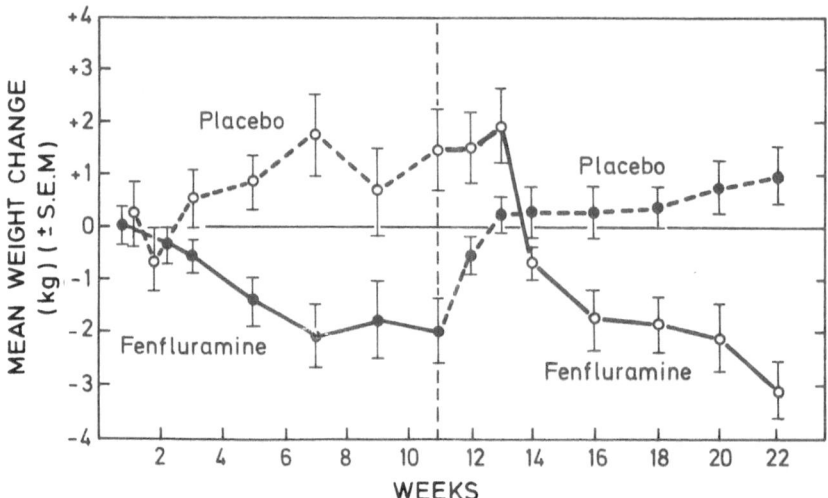

Figure 3   Weight loss and subsequent weight regain in a double-blind cross-over
study on patients treated initially with fenfluramine (from *Br. Med. J.* with
permission of the authors and the editor)

mazindol 1 mg per day in obese hypertensive patients was regained during
the ensuing 20-week cross-over placebo treatment[75] (see Figure 4). Weight

regain has also occurred following the cessation of treatment with biguanides and with thyroxine. Whether or not this reflects a metabolic adaptation or merely the development of drug tolerance, there is certainly no clinical evidence to support the assumption that any of the currently available anti-obesity agents will bring about a permanent change in energy balance. It follows that if a patient is unable to make such a change without the administration of a drug, there must be a high probability that weight regain will occur when the drug is discontinued.

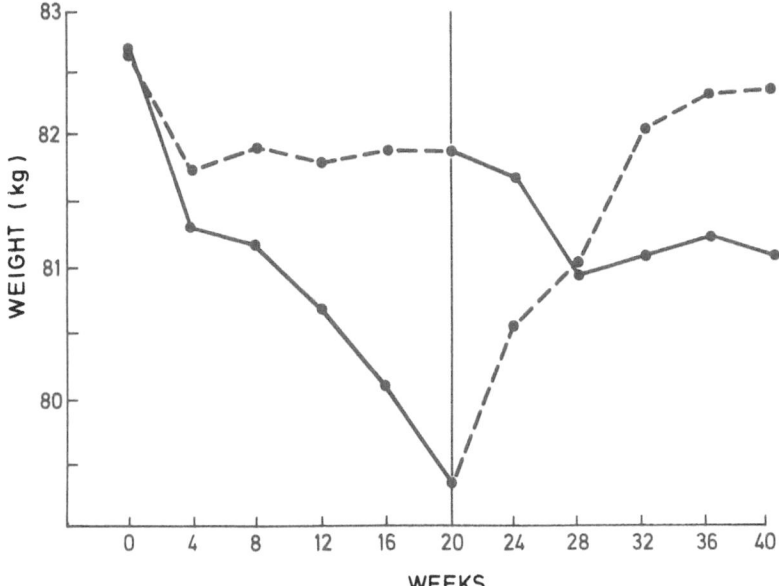

Figure 4   Mean weight loss and weight regain on a double-blind study of patients treated initially with mazindol. —— = drug therapy; – – – = treatment with placebo (by permission of the authors and editor of *Med. J. Aust.*)

Paradoxically, it is a common prescribing habit to recommend that drug therapy should be discontinued when weight loss ceases. It could thus be argued that the currently available agents should only be given if there is some short-term justification for weight loss. This could be medical – for example, to reduce before elective surgery – or psychological, for example, before a daughter's wedding. The British National Formulary go so far as to state that 'appetite-suppressant drugs have little place in the management of the obese patient and there is no substitute for will-power'[76].

LONG-TERM DRUG TREATMENT

It remains to be seen whether or not anti-obesity agents can occasionally be justified on a more long-term basis. This concept is contrary to present prescribing habit. In a recent review of 450 American physicians, 38% never used 'appetite-suppressants' and among those that did, only 25% would consider prescribing them for more than 12 weeks[77]. However, it seems possible that the price that must be paid to maintain the extra weight loss achieved by an anti-obesity agent is its indefinite administration. There are a few relatively anecdotal reports to suggest that such an approach might be effective, if 'effective' merely implies the prevention of weight regain as described in a 1-year study of fenfluramine[72]. Other studies include the 'successful' treatment of fifteen patients for periods of up to $2\frac{1}{2}$ years with maintenance doses of phentermine, after initial weight loss achieved using either D-amphetamine or phentermine itself[78]. Others have used diethylpropion with variable 'success'[79,80], while intermittent mazindol has been 'effective' in a small group of patients treated on average for 380 days[71]. It remains to be established whether or not the advantages that might accrue outweigh the potential risks of long-term therapy.

There is however a parallel between this concept and the current use of oral hypoglycaemic agents. The vast majority of insulin-independent diabetics can be controlled by appropriate dietary advice. Some, however, continue to have symptoms of such severity as would warrant administration of hypoglycaemic drugs. If the drug selected proves ineffective, it is discontinued. Otherwise, the dosage is adjusted until satisfactory control is established. That maintenance dosage is continued indefinitely unless the development of secondary failure necessitates future adjustments in treatment. It is possible that long-term treatment in the non-diabetic obese subject may prove of lasting value by preventing weight gain after effective weight loss. If this approach can be justified at all, its use should be restricted to those in whom the hazards of obesity are greatest.

SUMMARY AND CONCLUSIONS

1. Thyroxine is indicated in patients who are clinically or biochemically hypothyroid. The use of thyroid hormones, especially T_3, in the obese euthyroid subject, remains controversial and as yet unestablished.
2. The biguanides will improve glucose tolerance in diabetics without causing weight gain. Metformin is a valuable drug with which to treat diabetics who require oral hypoglycaemic therapy and are of normal or excess weight.
3. There is no evidence to support the popular contention that 'appetite-suppressant' drugs will help to establish normal eating habits. Indeed, the evidence would suggest that it is easier to maintain weight lost on diet alone than it is to maintain weight loss following drug treatment.
4. It follows that such drugs are not indicated unless appropriate dietary

treatment, with behavioural modification, has proved ineffective. Likewise, they should never be given except under careful medical supervision and as part of an overall management plan.

5. Fenfluramine, diethylpropion, phentermine and mazindol will all produce significant weight loss, the weight-reducing effect diminishing progressively. They are probably of comparable efficacy and are not without side-effects.

6. The individual response to such drugs is very variable. This may partly reflect differences in drug absorption and metabolism, and partly reflect the various metabolic adaptive changes that can occur in obesity; it may also reflect individual susceptibility to true drug tolerance.

7. Fenfluramine is a non-stimulant drug. It should be given continuously; the dose built up and reduced in a slow and stepwise manner to minimize the problems of side-effects.

8. The other 'appetite-suppressant' drugs are best given intermittently as this is as effective, cheaper and potentially safer.

9. The use of 'appetite-suppressant' drugs can be justified in carefully selected patients in whom there is a short-term justification for weight reduction. In the vast majority of such subjects, the extra weight lost that can be attributed to drug treatment will be regained once therapy is discontinued.

10. It remains to be established whether or not there is a place for the long-term use of 'appetite-suppressants', e.g. in preventing weight regain following radical medical treatment. This matter can only be resolved by careful long-term clinical evaluation.

11. It is regretted that, so far, we remain remarkably ignorant of the overall value of these drugs which have been prescribed so liberally and for so long.

References

1 Consumers Association (1978). *Which? Way to Slim.* (Portsmouth: Eyre and Spottiswoode Ltd.)
2 Connell, P. H. (1975). In M. N. G. Dukes (ed.). *Mylers Side Effects of Drugs*, vol. 8, p. 1. (Amsterdam–Oxford: Excerpta Medica)
3 Mackay, R. H. G. (1973). Long-term use of diethylpropion in obesity. *Curr. Med. Res. Opinion*, **8**, 489
4 Le Riche, W. H. and Csima, A. (1967). A long acting appetite suppressant drug. *Canad. Med. Assoc. J.*, **97**, 1016
5 Allen, G. S. (1977). A double blind clinical trial of diethylpropion hydrochloride, mazindol and placebo in the treatment of exogenous obesity. *Curr. Ther. Res.*, **22**, 678
6 McQuarrie, H. G. D. (1975). Clinical assessment of the use of an anorectic drug in a total weight reduction programme. *Curr. Ther. Res.*, **17**, 437

7 Bolding, P. T. (1974). Diethylpropion hydrochloride: an effective suppressant. *Curr. Ther. Res.*, **16**, 40

8 Nolan, G. R. (1975). Use of an anorexic drug in a total weight reduction program in prvate practice. *Curr. Ther. Res.*, **18**, 332

9 Stewart, D. A., Bailey, J. D. and Patell, H. (1970). Tenuate dospan as an appetite suppressant in the treatment of obese children. *App. Therapeut.*, 12, 34

10 Munro, J. F., McCuish, A. C., Wilson, E. M. and Duncan, L. J. P. (1968). Comparison in continuous and intermittent anorectic therapy in obesity. *Br. Med. J.*, **1**, 352

11 Campbell, C. J., Bhalla, I. P., Steele, H. M. and Duncan, L. J. P. (1977). A controlled trial of phentermine in obese diabetic patients. *Practitioner*, **218**, 851

12 Langlois, K. J., Forbes, J. A., Bell, C. W. and Grant, G. F. (Jr). (1974). A double blind clinical evaluation of the safety and efficacy of phentermine hydrochloride (fastin) in the treatment of exogenous obesity. *Curr. Ther. Res.*, **16**, 289

13 Truant, A. P., Lawrence, P. A. and Cobb, S. (1972). Phentermine resin as an adjunct in medical weight reduction: a controlled randomised double blind prospective study. *Curr. Ther. Res.*, **14**, 726

14 Moe, J. F. (1977). Phentermine hydrochloride therapy for exogenous obesity: an evaluation of interrupted therapy. *Curr. Ther. Res.*, **22**, 666

15 Harrison, L. C., King-Roach, A. P. and Sandy, K. C. (1975). Effects of mazindol on carbohydrate and insulin metabolism in obesity. *Metabolism*, **24**(12), 1353

16 Wallace, A. G. (1976). An 448 sandoz (mazindol) in the treatment of obesity. *Med. J. Aust.*, **1**, 343

17 Maclay, W. P. and Wallace, M. G. (1977). A multicentre general practice trial of mazindol in the treatment of obesity. *Practitioner*, **218**

18 Clinical trials: comparative merits of two weight reducing drugs (1978). (A report from the General Practice Research Group). *J. Pharmacotherapy*, **1**, 35

19 Bradley, M. J., Blum, N. J. and Scheib, R. K. (1974). Mazindol in obesity with known cardiac disease. *J. Int. Med. Res.*, **2**, 347

20 Bandisode, M. S. and Boshell, B. R. (1975). Double blind clinical evaluation of mazindol (42–558) in obese diabetics. *Curr. Ther. Res.*, **18**(6), 816

21 Schwartz, L. N. (1975). A non-amphetamine anorectic agent: preclinical background and a double blind clinical trial. *J. Int. Med. Res.*, **3**, 328

22 Heber, K. R. (1975). Double blind trial of mazindol in overweight patients. *Med. J. Aust.*, **2**, 566

23 Gomez, G. (1975). Obese patients in general practice: a comparison of the anorectic effects of mazindol, fenfluramine and placebo. *Clin. Trials J.*, **12**, 38

24 Smith, R. G., Innes, J. A. and Munro, J. F. (1975). Double blind evaluation of mazindol in refractory obesity. *Br. Med. J.*, **3**, 284

25 Sharma, R. K., Collipp, P. J., Rezvani, I., Strimas, J., Maddaiah, V. T. and Rezvani, E. (1973). Clinical evaluation of the anorexic activity and safety of 42–558 in children. *Clin. Pediat.*, **12**, 145

26 Allen G. S. (1977). A double blind clinical trial of diethylpropion hydrochloride, mazindol and placebo in the treatment of exogenous obesity. *Curr. Ther. Res.*, **22**, 678

27 Smith, D. E. (1974). A new anorexiant. *Rocky Mountain Med. J.*, **71**(1), 41

28 Sedgwick, J. P. (1975). Mazindol in the treatment of obesity. *Practitioner*, **214**, 418

29. Conte, A. (1973). Evaluation of sanorex – a new appetite suppressant. *Obesity/Bariatric Med.*, **2**, 104

30 Pinder, R. M., Brogden, R. N., Sawyer, P. R., Spreight, P. M. and Avery, G. S. (1975). Fenfluramine: A review of its pharmacological properties and therapeutic efficacy in obesity. *Drugs*, **10**(4), 241

31 Innes, J. A., Watson, M. L., Ford, M. J., Munro, J. F., Stoddart, M. E. and Campbell, D. B. (1977). Plasma fenfluramine levels, weight loss and side effects. *Br. Med. J.*, **2**, 1322

32 Doar, J. W. H., and Thomson, M. E. (1978). The influence of diet and fenfluramine on plasma sugar and insulin levels in patients with newly diagnosed maturity onset diabetes mellitus. *Curr. Med. Res. Opin.*, (in press)

33 Stowers, J. M. and Bewsher, P. D. (1969). Studies on the mechanism of weight reduction by phenformin. *Postgrad. Med. J.* (May Suppl.)

34 Cairns, A., Shalet, S., Marshall, A. J. and Hartog, M. (1977). A comparison of phenformin and metformin in the treatment of maturity onset obese diabetes. *Diabete et Metabolisme*, **3**, 183

35 Patel, D. P. and Stowers, J. M. (1964). Phenformin in weight reduction of obese diabetics. *Lancet*, **2**, 282

36 Clarke, B. F. and Duncan, L. J. P. (1968). Comparison of chlorpropamide and metformin treatment on weight and blood glucose response of uncontrolled obese diabetics. *Lancet* **1**, 123

37 Faludi, G., Chayes, Z. and Gerber, P. (1968). Rational treatment of the obese diabetic. *Postgrad. Med. J.*, **43**(21), 92

38 Lavieuville, M. and Isnard, F. (1975). Retrospective study of the cardiovascular fate of 190 diabetics treated for 5 years or more with biguanides alone. *Journees de Diabetologie Hotel-Dieu*, p.341

39 Mursky, S. and Schwartz. M. (1966). Phenformin diabetic control and body weight. *J. Mount Sinai Hosp.*, **33**(2), 180

40 Clarke, B. F. and Campbell, I. W. (1977). Comparison of metformin and chlorpropamide in non obese, maturity onset diabetics uncontrolled by diet. *Br. Med. J.*, **2**, 1576

41 Roginsky, M. S. and Barnett, J. (1966). Double blind study of phenethyl diguanide in weight control of obese nondiabetic subjects. *Am. J. Clin. Med.*, **19**(4), 223

42 Munro, J. F., MacCuish, A. C., Marshall, A., Wilson, E. M. and Duncan, L. J. P. (1969). Weight reducing effect of biguanides on obese non-diabetic women. *Br. Med. J.*, **2**, 13

43 Lawson, A. A. H., Strong, J. A., Roscoe, P. and Gibson, A. (1970). Comparisons of fenfluramine and metformin in treatment of obesity. *Lancet*, **1**, 437

44 Lutjens, A. and Smit, J. L. J. (1976). Effect of biguanide treatment in obese children. *Helv. Paediat. Acta*, **31**, 473

45 Miller, D. S. and Parsonage, S. (1975). Resistance to slimming; adaptation or illusion. *Lancet*, **1**, 773

46 Gwinup, G. and Poucher, R. (1967). A controlled study of thyroid analogs in the therapy of obesity. *Am. J. Med. Sci.*, **254**, 416

47 Bray, G. A. and Greenway, F. L. (1976). Pharmacological approaches to treating the obese patients. In M. J. Albrink (ed.), *Clinics in Endocrinology and Metabolism*, vol. 54, p.455. (London, Philadephia and Toronto: J. B. Saunders & Co. Ltd)

48 Kaplan, N. M. and Jose, A. (1970). A controlled study of thyroid analogs in the therapy of obesity. *Am. J. Med. Sci.*, **260**, 416

49 Hollingsworth, D. R., Amatruda, T. T. (Jr) and Scheig, R. (1970). Quantitative and qualitative effects of L-triiodithyrionine in massive obesity. *Metabolism*, **19**, 934

50 Asher, W. L. and Harper, M. W. (1973). Effect of human chorionic gonado-trophin on weight loss, hunger and feeling of well being. *Am. J. Clin. Nutr.*, **26**, 211

51 Hirsch, J. and Von Itallie, T. B. (1973)..The treatment of obesity. *Am. J. Clin. Nutr.*, **26**, 1039

52 Quaade, F. (1974). Untraditional treatment of obesity. In W. L. Burland, P. D. Samuel and J. Yudkin (eds). *Obesity*. (Edinburgh, London and New York: Churchill Livingstone)

53 Thorner, M. O., McNeilly, A. S., Hagan, C. and Besser, G. M. (1974). Long term treatment of galactorrhoea and hypogonadism with bronocriptine. *Br. Med. J.*, **2**, 419

54 Harrower, A. D. B., Yap, P. L., Nairn, I. M., Walton, H. J., Strong, J. A. and Craig, A. (1977). Growth hormone, insulin and prolactin secretion in anorexia nervosa and obesity during bromocriptine treatment. *Br. Med. J.*, **2**, 156

55 Quaade, F., Pakkenberg, H. and Juhl, E. (1974). Levo dopa as a treatment of obesity. *Acta Med. Scand.*, **195**, 129

56 Johanson, A. J. and Knorr, N. J. (1974). Treatment of anorexia nervosa by levo dopa. *Lancet*, **2**, 591

57 Scoville, B. A. (1973). Review of amphetamine-like drugs by the Food and Drug Administration. In G. A. Bray (ed.) *Obesity in Perspective*, p.441. (DHEW Publication No. (NIH) 75–707)

58 Seaton, D. A., Duncan, L. J. P. and Rose, K. (1961). Diethylproprion in the treatment of 'refractory' obesity. *Br. Med. J.*, **1**, 1009

59 Seaton, D. A., Rose, K. and Duncan, L. J. P. (1964a). A comparison of the appetitite suppressing properties of dexamphetamine and phentermine. *Scot. Med. J.*, **9**, 482

60 Seaton, D. A., Rose, K. and Duncan, L. J. P. (1964b). Sustained action chlorphentermine in the correction of refractory obesity. *Practitioner*, **193**, 698

61 Munro, J. F., Seaton, D. A. and Duncan, L. J. P. (1966). Treatment of refractory obesity with fenfluramine. *Br. Med. J.*, **2**, 624

62 Silverstone, J. R., Cooper, R. M. and Begg, R. R. (1970). A comparative trial of fenfluramine and diethylpropion in obesity. *Br. J. Clin. Pract.*, **24**(10)

63 Philips, B. L. D. (1977). Treatment of obesity: comparison of diethylpropion and fenfluramine. *Clin. Trials. J.*, **14**(2)

64 Follows, O. J. (1971). A comparative trial of fenfluramine and diethylpropion in obese, hypertensive patients. *Br. J. Clin. Pract.*, **25**, 5

65 Steel, J. M., Munro, J. F. and Duncan, L. J. P. (1973). A comparative trial of different regimes of fenfluramine and phentermine in obesity. *Practitioner*, **211**, 232

66 Stunkard, A., Rickels, K. and Hesbacher, P. (1973). Fenfluramine in the treatment of obesity. *Lancet*, **1**, 503

67 Vernace, B. J. (1974). Controlled comparative investigations of mazindol, D-amphetamine and placebo. *Obesity and Bariatric Med.*, **3**, 124

68 Kornhaber, A. (1973). Obesity-depression: clinical evaluation with a new anorexigenic agent. *Psychosomatics*, **14**, 162

69 Silverstone, T. (1974), Intermittent treatment with anorectic drugs. *Practitioner*, **212**, 245

70 Asher, W. L. (1978). Personal communication

71 Enzi, G., Baritussio, A., Machiori, E. and Crepaldi, G. (1976). Short term and long term clinical evaluation of non-amphetamine anorexiant (mazindol) in the treatment of obesity. *J. Int. Med. Res.*, **4,** 305

72 Hudson, K. D. (1977). The anorectic and hypotensive effect of fenfluramine in obesity. *J. Roy. Coll. of Gen. Pract.*, **27,** 497

73 Haugen, H. N. (1975). Double blind cross-over study of a new appetite suppressant. *Eur. J. Clin. Pharmacol.* **8,** 71

74 Carney, D. E. and Tweddell, E. D. (1975). Double blind evaluation of long acting diethylproprion hydrochloride in obese patients from a general practice. *Med. J. Aust.*, **1,** 13

75 Miach, P. J., Thomson, W., Doyle, A. E. and Louis, W. J. (1976). Double blind cross-over evaluation of mazindol in the treatment of obese hypertensive patients. *Med. J. Aust.*, **2,** 378

76 *British National Formulary* (1976–78) (England: Hazell Watson & Viney Ltd, Aylesbury, Bucks)

77 Lasagna, L. (1973). Attitudes towards appetite suppressants. *J. Am. Med. Assoc.*, **225,** 44

78 Smith, R. C. F. (1962). The long term control of obesity using sustained release appetite suppressants. *Br. J. Clin. Pract.*, **16,** 6

79 Craddock, D. (1973). *Obesity and its Management* (2nd edn). (London and New York: Churchill Livingstone)

80 Matthews, P. A. (1975). Diethylpropion in the treatment of obese patients seen in general practice. *Curr. Ther. Res.*, **17,** 340

5

The role of physical exercise in the management of obesity

P. Björntorp, L. Sjöström and L. Sullivan

INTRODUCTION

This chapter examines the value of physical training programmes in the prevention and management of obesity and its commonly associated conditions, including diabetes, hypertension and vascular disease. Physical exercise can be divided into two main types. One of these is largely static, engaging anaerobic pathways and muscle fibres of the white type rich in glycogen. Glucose is utilized and lactate is produced. The kind of athletic activity typical of this type of exercise is weight-lifting, short-distance running and wrestling. The other type of exercise is more dynamic; it involves the aerobic pathways and muscle fibres richer in aerobic enzymes and myoglobin. More fat substrate is utilized for energy purposes. The typical athletic activities here are the long-term, long-distance competitions, for example, running, swimming or cycling.

Physical exercise has a number of effects on different systems of the body, including the central and peripheral nervous system, circulation, hormones and metabolism of carbohydrate and fat; these effects vary at different times during a bout of physical exercise. Certain changes occur before the onset of exercise. During exercise pronounced changes occur, for example, in central and peripheral circulation. These and other changes, such as those affecting tissue metabolism and transport rates of energy, continue for some time after the end of exercise. Finally, after several bouts of exercise adaptive changes take place in the circulatory system, body composition and metabolism; these are the effects of physical training. They will be mainly considered because they constitute those changes which are of major significance with regard to the preventive and therapeutic effects of exercise on obesity.

THE EFFECT OF EXERCISE

Effects of exercise on body composition

The slimming effects of exercise are well-known. They are not necessarily synonymous with weight loss, particularly at the beginning of an exercise programme where muscle mass is built up to create a greater lean body mass than before exercise. The total amount of stored calories, however, will decrease from the start because the energy content of fat tissue is much higher than that of lean tissue even though the weight per unit of volume shows the opposite relationship.

Although this decrease in energy stores is obviously the result of a negative energy balance, the reason why exercise produces this is not fully understood. It seems probable that the effect of exercise is multifactorial, acting both on energy intake and energy expenditure. Mayer et al.[1] have described experiments and observations which suggest that exercise produces a decrease in energy intake leading to a reduction in weight. Stevenson et al.[2] in the rat, and Holm et al.[3] in man, have made similar obeservations after the first bouts of exercise in a training programme. There is still doubt as to whether or not this decrease in appetite occurs only immediately after the beginning of exercise sessions, or whether it continues throughout a training programme.

On the output side there is obviously an increase in energy expenditure during exercise; however from a therapeutic point of view the use of exercise as a treatment for obesity produces a rather depressing amount of weight loss per unit time of fairly hard work, even when large muscle groups are engaged. For example, the famous Vasa-loppet, an 85 km ski race, lasting some 6–10 h, for the non-athletic requires the energy equivalent of less than 1 kg of adipose tissue. Calculations of the energy expenditure during training programmes thus usually result in a suprisingly small net loss of calories, and a disappointingly small loss of weight due to the high energy value of adipose tissue. In practice the weight loss that occurs during such long-term training programmes cannot be explained entirely by the increased energy output caused by the work performed; some additional explanation is necessary. This may well be the effect on appetite regulation previously discussed, though the evidence for this remains inconclusive. There is, however, an alternative explanation. In addition to the energy requirements of direct external work there is also an energy need for 'basal' functions of the organism. These are usually referred to as non-shivering thermogenesis. There is considerable evidence that these energy-consuming reactions are of importance for the energy balance of the organism. It has even been argued that thermogenesis is the main regulatory factor for energy balance, and therefore possibly the main pathogenetic factor in obesity[4]. There is no doubt that thermogenesis is a significant factor in the overall energy balance although the detailed mechanism whereby it is regulated remains unknown. The site of such a regulating mechanism, although uncertain, is presumably one of the so-called 'futile cycles'. This is a phrase used to describe a series of metabolic events where heat is produced in an apparently wasteful way.

Recent evidence has been put forward that thermogenesis and thyroid hormones change in parallel, providing a possible basis for the explanation of the trigger mechanism for thermogenesis regulation. Thyroxine (T_4) is converted in the periphery into either 3,5,3'-triiodothyronine (T_3) which is the physiologically active form, or into another triiodinated hormone 3,5,3',-triiodothyronine (reverse T_3, RT_3) where the iodine atoms are situated differently. This latter hormone seems to be inactive. By changing the ratio of the conversion of T_4 to either T_3 or RT_3 the organism can thus alter the metabolic environment either to an energy-wasting or an energy-conserving situation. This can be exemplified by the decrease in T_3/RT_3 ratio during starvation, the increase during over-feeding, a decrease in a hot climate and an increase in a cold climate. (For review see Reference 5.) Recently the interrelationship between thyroid hormones function and physical exercise has been evaluated preliminarily in the rat. Thyroid hormone concentrations were measured in the plasma and their peripheral effectiveness examined on the lipolytic system of the epididymal fat pad *in vitro*. In comparison with pair-fed controls physical training caused only minor changes in thyroid-stimulating hormone (TSH) concentration following stimulation with thyroid-releasing hormone (TRH) and also in T_4, T_3 and RT_3 concentrations and peripheral sensitivity of T_3. In contrast, however, 24 h after one single exhaustive workload there was an increased T_3 over RT_3 ratio and furthermore an increased peripheral sensitivity to T_3 expressed as a larger lipolytic response to norepinephrine in the presence of T_3 *in vitro*. Another more striking change in thyroid hormone concentration and peripheral hormone response in this study was seen with age; older and fatter rats showing much lower T_3/RT_3 ratios and peripheral hormonal sensitivity, hypothetically associated with the increase in fat stores with age[6].

Obviously this study will have to be repeated with parallel measurements of energy expenditure. The results, however, are consistent with the hypothesis that the thyroid hormones and thermogenesis are involved in the regulation of the energy stores of the body during a physical training programme. It seems possible that during the start of an exercise programme thermogenesis is increased by changes in thyroid hormone metabolism causing a decrease in body fat. The known stability of the body fat stores, and the apparently perfect energy balance in well-trained subjects, such as endurance athletes[7] is consistent with thyroid hormone concentration returning to the 'normal' steady-state concentration. Such a mechanism, which is supported by these experimental data, would help to explain the missing energy expenditure that occurs at the beginning of an exercise programme and which cannot be accounted for by the work alone, or perhaps by possible changes in the energy intake.

The decreasing effect of exercise on body fat is apparently not invariable. In hyperplastic obese subjects, characterized by severe enlargement of adipose tissue with an elevated number of fat cells, several studies have shown that exercise produces a slower than normal reduction[8], or no decrease[9] or even an increase[10] of body fat during a training programme on *ad libitum* diet. In its pronounced form this is a rare condition compared with the normal response in moderate obesity[11]; it apparently constitutes an exception from the general rule that body fat decreases with physical training. There is no obvious explanation why some grossly overweight subjects fail to reduce their body fat during physical training. Indeed, the expenditure of energy by work of these patients would, if anything, be greater than that of a non-obese or moderately obese subject, simply because their severe obesity requires extra energy to support their body during exercise. Possibly they do not regulate their appetite normally during exercise programmes, though dietary histories reveal no obvious deviations[12]. Finally, the hypothetical thyroid regulation mechanism mentioned above might be an additional possibility.

From a practical point of view one might ask how much exercise is needed in order to produce a significant change in body fat stores. Unfortunately, neither the type nor the duration of exercise required is precisely known. Clearly, the longer the duration and the heavier the intensity of the programme, the more fat will be lost. As a general rule, however, it has been found that an exercise programme consisting of three sessions per week, each of about 45 min at a work intensity approximately equal to that of jogging, produces an average weight loss of 0·5 kg per month without any recommendations concerning the diet[13].

Changes in metabolism by exercise

Physical training causes several changes in metabolism. One of the earliest, and possibly the most pronounced, is the decrease in plasma insulin, either during fasting or during a glucose challenge[14]. The effect of exercise on plasma insulin occurs in the absence of changes in body fat, as illustrated both during training programmes of those hyperplastic obese subjects who fail to lose weight and after a single bout of exercise[3,10]. It follows that the effect cannot be attributed to the fact that exercise usually diminishes body fat and would appear to be the result of the exercise itself. The reason for the decrease in plasma insulin is unknown. Several possibilities have been considered, but none is a satisfactory explanation. These include changes in plasma amino acid concentration[15], changes in some of the hormones with an effect opposite to that of insulin[12], and a decrease in the glucose challenge of the β-cell[10]. Cortisol secretion seems to diminish, but whether this is a primary effect of training causing a decrease of plasma insulin, or a secondary effect of the insulin decrease, is not known. The decrease is apparently due both to decreased secretion and, to some extent, an increased insulin removal[16]. A further explanation of the decrease in insulin secretion is the known insulin-like effect of muscle contraction[17] possibly providing a synergistic effect to insulin and there-fore by feedback mechanisms a decreased secretion from the pancreas. Nervous system adaptations influencing the insulin secretion seem to be another possibility not as yet examined.

In addition to the insulin-like activity found in muscle after contraction, there remains the possibility that physical training causes a more long-lasting, 'chronic' adaptation with an increased insulin sensitivity of muscle. At present the evidence for this is only indirect but nevertheless suggestive. Non-diabetic patients with intermittent claudication have been found to have not only the same type of enzymic adaptations in the muscle tissue distal to the arterial constriction as well-trained subjects, but also a plasma insulin concentration which is as low as that of well-trained subjects. The plasma insulin concentrations are inversely related to the amount of muscle mass subjected to ischaemia, suggesting a role for the adapted muscle in the regulation of plasma insulin concentration[18]. Recent more direct observations suggest that the adapted muscle is indeed more insulin-sensitive because at the same insulin concentration the glucose uptake is increased in the leg of the patient with intermittent claudication both during basal conditions[19] and after infusion of glu-cose[20]. It may well be that the physically trained muscle shows the same type of adaptation, and this may then provide the reason for the low plasma insulin concentration.

Plasma triglycerides are also lowered by physical training[21] and after acute physical work[21,22], an effect independent of possible changes in food intake by exercise[23]. It seems possible that this effect is secondary to the decrease in plasma insulin because the concentrations of plasma insulin and triglycerides are interdependent[24]. In addition, particularly after acute work, it may be that plasma triglycerides are extracted more rapidly from the plasma for energy-producing purposes during work, resulting in a decreased plasma concentration.

Glucose tolerance is far less affected by training than are plasma insulin and triglyceride concentrations. There is, however, a demonstrable effect, possibly parallel to the decrease in body fat[25].

The effects of exercise on blood pressure
Several haemodynamic effects of physical training are demonstrable.

These include a decrease in cardiac output at a given submaximal work-load, presumably compensated for in the exercising muscles by an increased efficiency of the enzymic apparatus to extract available oxygen in the blood flowing through the working muscle[26]. Early hypertension is characterized by an increase in cardiac output, while an increase in peripheral resistance seems to be a later phenomenon. It is therefore logical that physical training should decrease the elevated blood pressure in mild hypertension by decreasing the elevated cardiac output. That this is indeed the case has been demonstrated, albeit in a small series[27].

The recent observation in a non-selected, total population of mild hypertension that body fat, fat cell size, plasma insulin and triglycerides are elevated and glucose tolerance decreased[28] has interesting implications for the pathogenesis, prevention and therapy of early hypertension. One might speculate that there may be a common denominator for the metabolic derangement and the hypertension and the associated hypertrophic obesity. Physical training tends to normalize all these variables; likewise dietary treatment with calorie restriction, but without changing the salt intake, also decreases blood pressure effectively[29], reduces the degree of obesity, diminishes plasma insulin and triglyceride concentrations and improves glucose tolerance. This suggests that there may be a large aetiological overlap between hypertrophic obesity, endogenous hyper-triglyceridaemia, adult-onset diabetes mellitus and essential hypertension. That all these conditions are improved by physical training, and/or by weight loss brought about by dietary restriction, must suggest that there are significant common pathogenic factors.

PREVENTIVE AND THERAPEUTIC ASPECTS

It has been seen that physical training will indeed decrease body fat by a reduction in fat cell size[7]. It has also been shown that physical training decreases plasma insulin and triglycerides and improves, to some extent, glucose tolerance. It is thus logical to consider physical training as a means of treating or preventing those conditions characterized by these abnormalities. The corresponding disease entities are hypertrophic obesity with hyperinsulinaemia, endogenous hypertriglyceridaemia, and adult-onset diabetes mellitus. Physical exercise may be of particular value in subjects suffering from a combination of these conditions. It has already been demonstrated that it is possible to treat hypertrophic obesity with physical training. Although improvement of glucose tolerance and reduction of plasma triglycerides also occur, there are no clinical trials which have evaluated the efficacy of physical training as a therapeutic alternative in these conditions compared with the use of diet or drugs. One study, currently under way, would suggest that the therapeutic value of exercise in diabetic patients requiring treatment with a sulphonylurea is variable.

The possibility of treating early hypertension and its associated metabolic derangements has already been mentioned. It should be stressed that the value of exercise as an alternative form of treatment for this common disorder requires to be further evaluated. There are other potential preventive and therapeutic implications of physical training. These include its use in various forms of vascular disease, another condition frequently found in association with obesity. It has been shown that angina pectoris improves after physical training[30]. This effect was probably obtained by the decrease in heart work at a defined submaximal workload[30]. It seems plausible that the enzymic adaptation in the periphery in the trained muscle, associated with a decreased local blood flow, enables the muscle cell to extract the available oxygen from the blood more efficiently. In this way the peripheral adaptation of the working muscle takes over some of the responsibility for its own oxygen supply, permitting exercise to be undertaken at a lower cardiac output. This reduces the demand of the myocardium for oxygen at a defined work-load and can therefore prevent attacks of angina pectoris. There is of course the alternative possibility that a training programme will result in an increased collateral circulation in the myocardium, an effect that has been demonstrated in trained dogs following arterial ligation[31].

Intermittent claudication is another clinical entity of considerable interest. Physical training produces an improvement in such patients by increasing the walking distance before the onset of pain. This can be attributed to an adaptation of the muscle cells with increased activities of several enzymes in anaerobic and aerobic pathways[32]. It seems likely that these changes enhance the ability of the working muscle to extract oxygen from the available blood, the supply of which has been reduced by arterial restriction. It should be noted that these enzyme activities are increased even before supervised physical training has begun[32]. This may be due to the fact that the 'trigger' mechanism for enzyme adaptation is more active due to the restricted blood flow. The nature of this 'trigger' is unknown.

There are at present insufficient data to indicate whether or not physical training programmes are of any value in the primary prevention of myocardial infarction. Those few fully controlled studies that have been reported have dealt mainly with the problem of secondary prevention by physical training. The results in this important field are so far also inconclusive. One difficulty has been the high dropout rate that occurs during training programmes. In one study this amounted to 70% of subjects after 3 years. At the end of this study there was no significant difference between the trained group and the controls[33]. In another study of a different design a significant difference was, however, found[34] and here the dropout frequency was more moderate.

The following points should be remembered: physical training reduces several known risk factors for myocardial infarction such as early hypertension, hypertriglyceridaemia, diabetes mellitus, physical inactivity and obesity; furthermore, it may encourage the individual subject to give up smoking. Thus training can improve most of the non-hereditary risk factors for myocardial infarction, though some of these factors are relatively minor. The risk factors not affected include hypercholesterolaemia and established hypertension; the effect on smoking is indirect and uncertain. To date controlled studies of relatively limited duration have failed to show any striking effect on survival and reinfarction. It seems possible, however, that within the total population of patients suffering from myocardial infarcts there will be certain sub-groups more likely to benefit from training programmes because the major risk factors in these particular patients can be improved by exercise. An additional benefit of training in all patients is the psychological reassurance provided by the patient's own observation that exercise is still possible after myocardial infarction[33]. There are other psychological benefits associated with physical training which should not be overlooked. Tension-relieving effects are often reported, and it is possible that there is less absenteeism, due to an improvement in general health, although the studies of this nature require further careful evaluation.

It must also be remembered that physical training is not without risk. The main danger is cardiovascular. Sudden deaths have been reported in untrained persons starting an exercise programme too enthusiastically and at too high an initial degree of activity. A health check is advisable in sedentary middle-aged people before commencing strenuous exercise. Professional supervision is also advisable. Physical exertion during infection may be dangerous. These rare but serious side-effects should be avoided with appropriate selection and supervision. Locomotor damage to tendons, joints and muscles at the beginning of training programmes can also be minimized if professional supervision is provided, ensuring a slow start. Generally, it seems likely that the side-effects of physical training appropriately performed are less frequent and less serious than the side-effects of drug therapy in those conditions in which physical training seems effective.

FEASIBILITY OF PHYSICAL TRAINING PROGRAMMES

Any form of long-term treatment is only of value if it is sufficiently acceptable to ensure a reasonable degree of patient compliance. At first glance there are obvious difficulties with physical training programmes. A high proportion of patients, even those most highly motivated like subjects who have suffered a myocardial infarction, will drop out of a programme after a few years[33]. There are other similar discouraging reports. In spite of maximal efforts to keep obese subjects in training programmes the drop-out frequency is about 30%[8-10,12,13]. Further analysis of the problem reveals several important factors which contribute to the degree of adherence to a programme. Bjurö[35] has studied randomly selected middle-aged men of sedentary habit. He has found that initial resistance to the programme was responsible for the largest number of non-participants. The number of people who refuse to participate naturally depends on their age, mode of selection and motivation. Among those men who actually start a programme further dropout can be minimized by various measures. These include ensuring that the participants are provided with thorough initial information about the nature and purpose of the programme. The further feedback information concerning each participant's degree of fitness, body weight, blood lipids, etc. throughout the programme is also essential as it acts as an incentive and encourages subjects to continue with the programme. Other measures include the attendance of a coach at most of the training sessions. Furthermore, outdoor exercises are more attractive than artificial indoor exercise machines.

SPECIAL PROBLEMS IN PHYSICAL TRAINING OF OBESE SUBJECTS

Numerous studies have shown that obese people have difficulty in achieving and maintaining a high work-load[36-38]. The reason for this may be that in obese individuals heavy physical exercise activates several different pathophysiological mechanisms which, separately or together, limit the cardiopulmonary capacity. There seems to be a correlation between obese individuals' subjective experience of physical training and pathophysiological reactions, even at relatively low work-loads[37,39]. Some of these reactions will be discussed below.

High energy costs

The mere process of transporting excess weight when rising to the erect position and walking at an even pace entails extra muscular work. Likewise exercises used in heavy physical training also involve this additional energy expenditure for weight support and body stabilization. This is accentuated by vigorous, uneven movements. In absolute terms, heavy physical exercise in the obese yields a low external output in relation to the costs, and a high level of heat generation. The increased heat generation in the obese requires to be balanced by corresponding heat expenditure with the same precise temperature regulation as in the non-obese. There are, however, several factors that may result in a poorer capacity for the obese to dissipate heat. Adipose tissue contains small amounts of water and is a poor heat conductor[40]. Pronounced rotundity also results in a low area-to-volume ratio for heat dissipation. The density of thermally activated sweat-glands is also lower than in normal individuals[41].

When the thermal homeostasis fails in obese subjects due to a higher heat load of exercise than can be regulated, the blood flow is redistributed increasingly from the working musculature to the periphery in order to facilitate heat dissipation. The elevated core body temperature leads to tachycardia, hyperventilation and increased blood pressure, eventually causing extreme discomfort and an inability to continue working. This may even result in fatalities among young and otherwise healthy individuals with large body size[42], when their heat acclimatization is poor and the capacity to dissipate heat is further compromised by high environmental temperature.

Defective pulmonary function

Pulmonary function in obesity seems to exhibit certain pathological characteristics that are related to the degree of adiposity[39]. The additional fat mass results in an increase in respiratory work and a raised metabolic cost of respiration[43-45]. In extreme obesity the fat mass produces an increased intra-abdominal pressure, reduced expiratory reserve volume and reduced lung compliance. Some obese subjects exhibit different degrees of arterial hypoxia which has been related to uneven alveolar ventilation and perfusion[39,46].

Unlike normal individuals, obese subjects also experience dyspnoea at submaximal work-loads[39]. The obese subject unconsciously chooses a respiratory pattern which probably represents an attempt to avoid high elastic strains during the inspiratory phase of respiration. This is accomplished by hyperventilating at a high respiratory rate and low tidal volume[45,47]. We have observed obese patients adopting this respiratory pattern when exercising on a bicycle ergometer with gradual increase of the resistance and experiencing some discomfort at relatively low loads. We have also found that these patients abandon this respiratory pattern after fitness training, in spite of not losing weight. However, the well-known Pickwickian syndrome (hypoventilation, hypercapnoea, periodic respiration, somnolence, polycythaemia, cyanosis, elevated pressure in the pulmonary artery and hypertrophy and failure of the right ventricle) is considered to be extremely rare even in patients with very pronounced obesity[48]. Certainly no correlation has been found between degree of hypercapnoea and the severity of obesity. Likewise, isolated hypertrophy of the right ventricle has not been demonstrated in systematic post-mortem studies of obese subjects[49].

Physical inactivity in the obese is naturally more likely to become permanent if there are other conditions present which may also restrict activity, such as osteoarthrosis and obstructive airways disease[50]. In these circumstances it may be difficult to find any form of activity that produces a sufficiently great increase in exercise without aggravating the patient's other symptoms.

Cardiovascular dysfunction

In a series of studies in obese subjects, Alexander *et al.* have demonstrated various haemodynamic abnormalities. These include an increased cardiac output and increased blood volume in order to supply the large body fat mass[48,51,52]. These abnormalities disappeared after weight reduction[53]. Certain other pathophysiological characteristics, such as high pulmonary artery pressure, increased filling pressure in the left ventricle during light exercise and hypertrophy of the left ventricle, were not reversible during an observation period of up to 3 years after weight loss[53].

The elevated heart load found in obesity during even light work might increase during hard physical training, and possibly produce unwanted or even dangerous effects. Although this risk is not easy to prove, it seems pertinent to respect the patient's reports of discomfort and modulate the training programme accordingly[38]. This may be particularly important when treating elderly and extremely obese patients.

DESIGN OF PHYSICAL TRAINING PROGRAMMES FOR OBESE SUBJECTS

Screening procedures

There are good reasons for taking a careful history and thoroughly examining potential candidates for physical training before drawing up a detailed exercise programme. Previous diseases or injuries, such as periodic back ailments and recurrent sports injuries from previous active periods, should be carefully evaluated and drug medication should be considered.

When selecting patients for physical training and designing an exercise programme it is usually important to know which factor or factors limit the patient's physical capacity – muscular, cardiac, pulmonary or other factors. Depending on the exact pattern of the training the pre-training clinical evaluation will vary, but certain metabolic, cardiovascular and haemodynamic measurements should be made. We routinely determine insulin resistance, glucose tolerance and blood lipid concentrations. We also use exercise tests very liberally, with a stepwise increase of the load, to determine capacity (VO$_2$max and VO$_2$max/kg body weight). The blood pressure reaction up to maximal load is registered. A chest X-ray is taken routinely. Recent advances in non-invasive methods for cardiac diagnoses will be valuable when more generally available.

Motivation-promoting measures

The motivation of patients and composition of training programmes require further systematic study. The principles and practical guidelines put forward here are based on our own experience, and mainly relate to controlled training programmes performed for research purposes.

Patients who remain in the study after clinical examination must be given the necessary time to prepare for the training programme. Repeated information meetings over a period of a couple of months have been found suitable in several studies. During these introductory meetings, which are held at the same times as the subsequent training sessions, the patients are given information about the various known effects of physical training and the special problems obese individuals have to cope with when undertaking such a programme. The effects of prolonged submaximal exercise are explained, e.g. increased combustion of fat stores and increase of muscle mass, increased insulin sensitivity in peripheral tissues, lowered insulin concentration, lowered cardiac work during submaximal exercise and better oxygen transport, a certain metabolic adaptation in the working muscles, lower plasma lipid levels and possibly a reduced risk of diabetes mellitus and atherosclerotic diseases. During the motivation process, we also discuss those pathophysiological factors which make it particularly difficult for untrained obese individuals to endure prolonged submaximal work. We emphasize that most of these factors diminish with weight loss and improved physical fitness. If hyperplastic patients are to participate in the training programme without dieting, we tell them that it is doubtful whether the treatment will reduce their weight, but highly probable that it will improve their metabolic abnormalities. Warnings about the increased risks of direct training injuries, such as sprains etc., in untrained obese people with unreliable body stability have probably been of value, not only for prevention but also for helping the patients cope with injuries when they have occurred.

We also explain the difference between physical performance during weight-supported work, e.g. on a bicycle ergometer (VO$_2$max) and performance during movement from one location to another (VO$_2$max/kg body weight). Improvement of the latter factor is of greater practical importance, and can of course be achieved both by increasing oxygen uptake and by weight reduction.

After a series of general information meetings the patients should ideally receive further detailed information in smaller training groups, with not more than five patients in each group. The additional information will depend upon the level of physical fitness (VO_2max/kg body weight) in the sub-group, and the estimated margin for training effects. At every stage, before and during training, we appeal to the patients to attend regularly and to stimulate and encourage each other to stick to the regimen. The duration and details of the programme, and the routine medical tests that will be carried out, should be agreed with the patients in advance and each participant should be given a complete schedule.

The training programme

Little is known about how a physical training programme for obese patients should be designed in order to achieve the desired effects in the individual case. It would seem quite clear, however, that relatively prolonged submaximal exercise should have the best effect on combustion of storage fat. The most suitable frequency, intensity and composition of the training sessions needs, however, to be established by comparative studies, taking age, primary physical fitness, muscle fibre composition, and the type and degree of metabolic abnormality into consideration. In the absence of conclusive studies on these points, we have drawn conclusions empirically from our own experience.

When relatively hard, structured training programmes are carried out, comprehensive dynamic and static muscle training, alternating with short periods of cardiopulmonary fitness training, probably represents a more easily tolerated form of energy expenditure than equal expenditure from running and jogging alone. In the initial phase of a training programme, these patients seem to experience more discomfort from exercises entailing movement of body weight, e.g. step-tests, than in weight-supported exercises giving the same heart rate, e.g. on a bicycle ergometer. A finding of a normal and better-than-normal exercise capacity during weight-supported exercise is often encouraging for the obese patient. The obese often have a large body cell mass and high working capacity when not transporting their own weight. With improving physical fitness, patients often seem to become more interested in non-supported exercises, and further stimulation has been reported when the programme has contained a great variety of exercises of this type, e.g. circle training with jogging, skipping, rhythmic dancing, step-tests etc. Limiting the programme to a few pieces of apparatus, such as lifting weights, pedalling a bicycle ergometer and rowing on a rowing machine, has been found to reduce the patient's motivation. Some form of graded exercise in which the patient can himself gauge his performance may favourably be included in each training session. The patients can then compete among themselves and with their own previous results.

One factor which may have helped patients to complete the treatment is that we always appeal to them to report unavoidable absence in advance and to consult the physician in charge of the training if they become ill or suffer injury. In return, we promise them medical attention, even in their homes if necessary, in the event of intercurrent diseases, as well as offering transport by private car to and from the training sessions in the event of temporary transport problems.

References

1 Mayer, J., Marshall, N. B., Vitale, J. J., Christensen, J. H., Mashayekhi, M. B. and Stare, F. J. (1954). Exercise, food intake and body weight in normal rats and genetically obese adult mice. *Am. J. Physiol.*, **177,** 544

2 Stevenson, J. A. F., Box, B. M., Feleki, V. and Beaton, J. R. (1966). Bouts of exercise and food intake in the rat. *J. Appl. Physiol.*, **21,** 118

3 Holm, G., Björntorp, P. and Jagenburg, R. (1978). Effects on carbohydrate lipid and amino acid metabolism during the days following submaximal physical exercise in man. *J. Appl. Physiol.* **44,** 128

4 Miller, D. S. (1974). Thermogenesis in every day life. Proc. Sec. Congr. of Energy Balance in Man. *Excerpta Medica*, p. 94

5 Westgren, U. (1976). On the production of thyroxine, active and inactive triiodothyronine in man. Thesis. Studentlitteratur, Lund, Sweden

6 Wirth, A., Holm. B., Lindstedt, G. and Björntorp, P. (1978). Thyroid hormones in the physically trained rat. *J. Appl. Physiol.* (in press)

7 Björntorp. P., Grimby, G., Sanne, H., Sjöström, L., Tibblin, G. and Wilhelmsen, L. (1972). Adipose tissue fat cell size in relation to metabolism in weightstabile, physically active men. *Horm. Metab. Res.*, **4,** 182

8 Björntorp, P., de Jounge, K., Krotkiewski, M., Sullivan, L., Sjöström, L. and Stenberg, J. (1973). Physical training in human obesity. III. Effects of long-term physical training on body composition. *Metabolism*, **22,** 1467.

9 Björntorp, P., de Jounge, K., Sjöström, L. and Sullivan, L. (1973). Physical training in human obesity. II. Effects on plasma insulin in glucose-intolerant subjects without marked hyperinsulinemia. *Scand. J. Clin. Lab. Invest.*, **32,** 41

10 Björntorp, P., de Jounge, K., Sjöström, L. and Sullivan, L. (1970). The effect of physical training on insulin production in obesity. *Metabolism*, **19,** 631

11 Larsson, B. (1978). Obesity. A population study of men with special reference to development and consequences for the health. Thesis. Gotab, Kungälv, Sweden

12 Björntorp, P., Holm, G., Jacobsson, B., Schiller-de Jounge, K., Lundberg, P-A., Sjöström, L., Smith, U. and Sullivan, L. (1977). Physical training in human hyperplastic obesity. IV. Effects on the hormonal status. *Metabolism*, **26,** 319

13 Krotkiewski, M., Sjöström, L. and Sullivan, L. (1977). Effects of long-term training on adipose tissue cellularity and body composition in hypertrophic and hyperplastic obesity. *Int. J. Obesity*, (Abstract) **2,** 395

14 Björntorp, P., Fahlén, M., Grimby, G., Gustafson, A., Holm, J., Renström, P. and Scherstén, T. (1972). Carbohydrate and lipid metabolism in middle-aged, physically well-trained men. *Metabolism*, **21,** 1037

15 Holm, G., Sullivan, L., Jagenburg, R. and Björntorp, P. (1978). Effects of physical training and lean body mass on plasma amino acids in man. *J. Appl. Physiol.*, **44,** 342

16 Wirth, A., Holm, G., Nilsson, B., Smith, U. and Bjorntorp, P. (1978). Insulin kinetics and insulin binding to adipocytes in physically trained and food-

restricted rats (submitted for publication)

17 Holloszy, J. O. and Narahara, H. T. (1965). Studies of tissue permeability. X. Changes in permeability to 3-methylglucose associated with contraction of isolated frog muscle. *J. Biol. Chem.*, **240**, 3493

18 Holm, J., Dahllöf, A-C., Björntorp, P. and Schersten, T. (1973). Glucose tolerance, plasma insulin, and lipids in intermittent claudication with reference to muscle metabolism. *Metabolism*, **22**, 1395

19 Hammarsten, J., Holm, J., Björntorp, P. and Schersten, T. (1977). Glucose tolerance and fractional extraction of glucose and insulin in patients with peripheral arterial insufficiency. Effect of arterial reconstructive surgery. *Metabolism*, **26**, 883

20 Hammarsten, J. and Schersten, T. (1978). Personal communication

21 Holloszy, J. O., Skinner, J. S., Toro, G. and Cureton, T. K. (1964). Effects of a six month program of endurance exercise on the serum lipids of middle-aged men. *Am. J. Cardiol.*, **14**, 753

22 Carlson, L. A. and Mossfeldt, F. (1964). Acute effects of prolonged, heavy exercise on the concentration of plasma lipids and lipoproteins in man. *Acta Physiol. Scand.*, **62**, 51

23 Gyntelberg, F., Rennie, M. J., Hickson, R. C. and Holloszy, J. O. (1977). Effect of training on the response of plasma glucagon to exercise, *J. Appl. Physiol.*, **43**, 302

24 Reaven, G. M., Lerner, R. L., Stern, M. P., Farquhar, J. W. and Nakaniski, R. (1967). Role of insulin in hypertriglyceridemia. *J. Clin. Invest.*, **11**, 1756

25 Björntorp, P., Berchtold, P., Grimby, G., Lindholm, B., Sanne, H., Tibblin, G. and Wilhelmsen, L. (1972). Effects of physical training on glucose tolerance, plasma insulin and lipids and on body composition in men after myocardial infarction. *Acta. Med. Scand.*, **192**, 439

26 Varnauskas, E., Björntorp, P., Fahlén, M., Prerovsky, I. and Stenberg, J. (1970). Effects of physical training on exercise blood flow and enzymatic activity in skeletal muscle. *Cardiovascular Res.*, **4**, 418

27 Sannerstedt, T., Wasir, H., Henning, R. and Werkö, L. (1973). Systemic haemodynamics in mild arterial hypertension before and after physical training. *Clin. Sci. Mole. Med.*, **45**, 145

28 Berglund, G., Larsson, B., Andersson, O., Larsson, O., Svärdsudd, K., Björntorp, P. and Wilhelmsen, L. (1976). Body composition and glucose metabolism in hypertensive middle-aged males. *Acta. Med. Scand.*, **200**, 163

29 Reisin, E., Abel, R., Modan, M., Silverberg, D. S., Eliahou, H. E. and Modan, B. (1978). Effect of weight loss without salt restriction on the reduction of blood pressure in overweight hypertensive patients. *N. Engl. J. Med.*, **298**, 1

30 Varnauskas, E., Bergman, H., Houk, P. and Björntorp, P. (1966). Haemodynamic effects of physical training in coronary patients. *Lancet*, **2**, 8

31 Sanne, H. and Sivertsson, R. (1968). The effect of exercise on the development of collateral circulation after experimental occlusion of the femoral artery in the cat. *Acta Physiol. Scand.*, **73**, 257

32 Holm, J., Dahllöf, A-G., Björntorp, P. and Schersten, T. (1973). Enzyme studies in muscles of patients with intermittent claudication. Effect of training. *Scand. J. Clin. Lab. Invest.*, **31**, 201

33 Sanne, H. (1973). Exercise tolerance and physical training of non-selected patients after myocardial infarction. Thesis. *Acta. Med. Scand.* (Suppl. 557)

34 Palatsi, J. (1976). Feasibility of physical training after myocardial infarction and its effect on return to work, morbidity and mortality. Thesis. *Acta Med. Scand.* (Suppl. 599)

35 Bjurö, T. (1978). Personal communication

36 Dempsey, J. A. (1964). Anthropometrical observations on obese and non-obese young men undergoing a program of vigorous physical exercise. *Res. Quart.*, **35**, 275

37 Kenrick, M. M., Ball, M. F. and Canary, J. J. (1972). Exercise and weight reduction in obesity. *Arch. Phys. Med.*, **53**, 323

38 Björntorp, P., de Jounge, K., Sjöström, L. and Sullivan, L. (1973). Physical training in human obesity. II. Effects on plasma insulin in glucose-intolerant subjects without marked hyperinsulinemia. *Scand. J. Clin. Lab. Invest.*, **32**, 41

39 Dempsey, J. A. and Rankin, J. (1967). Physiologic adaptations of gas transport systems to muscular work in health and disease. *Am. J. Phys. Med.*, **46**, 582

40 Buskirk, E. R., Bar-Or, O. and Kollias, J. (1969). Physiological effects of heat and cold. In N. J. Wilson (ed.), *Obesity*, p. 119 (Philadelphia: F. A. Davis Co.)

41 Bar-Or, O., *et al.* (1968). Distribution of heat activated sweat glands in obese and lean men and women. *Hum. Biol.*, **40**, 233

42 Fox, B. L., Matthews, O. K. Kaufman, W. S. and Bowers, R. W. (1966). Effects of football equipment on thermal balance and energy cost during exercise. *Res. Quart. Am. Assoc. Health Phys. Educ.*, **37**, 332

43 Naimark, A. and Cherniack, R. M. (1960). Compliance of the respiratory system and its components in health and obesity. *J. Appl. Physiol.*, **15**, 377

44 Sharp, J. T., Henry, J. P., Sweany, S. K., Meadows, W. R. and Pietras, R. J. (1964). The total work of breathing in normal and obese men. *J. Clin. Invest.*, **43**, 728

45 Dempsey, J. A., Reddan, W., Rankin, J. and Balke, B. (1966). Alveolar to arterial gas exchange during muscular work in obesity. *J. Appl. Physiol.*, **21**, 1807

46 Holley, H. S., Milic-Emili, J., Bechlake, M. R. and Bates, D. V. (1967). Regional distribution of pulmonary ventilation and perfusion on obesity. *J. Clin. Invest.*, **46**(4), 475

47 Turrell, D. T., Austin, R. C. and Alexander, J. K., (1964). Cardio-respiratory responses of very obese subjects to treadmill exercise. *J. Lab. Clin. Invest.*, **64**, 107

48 Alexander, J. K., Amad, K. H. and Cale, V. W. (1962). Observations on some clinical features of extreme obesity, with particular reference to cardio-respiratory effects. *Am. J. Med.*, **32**, 512

49 Amad, K. H., Brennan, J. C. and Alexander, J. K. (1965). The cardiac pathology of chronic exogenous obesity. *Circulation*, **32**, 740

50 Bedell, G. N., Wilson, W. R. and Seebohm, P. M. (1958). Pulmonary function in obese persons. *J. Clin. Invest.*, **37**, 1049

51 Alexander, J. K., Dennis, E. W., Smith, W. G., Amad, K. H., Duncan, W. C. and Austin, R. C. (1962). Blood volume, cardiac output and distribution of systemic blood flow in extreme obesity. *Cardiovasc. Res. Center Bull.*, 1 (Suppl. II), 39

52 Alexander, J. K. (1964). Obesity and cardiac performance. *Am. J. Cardiol.*, **14** 860

53 Alexander, J. K. and Peterson, K. L. (1972). Cardiovascular effects of weight reduction. *Circulation*, **45**, 310

54 Sjöström, L. Björntorp, P. and Vrana, J. (1971). Microscopic fat cell size measurements on frozen-cut adipose tissue in comparison with automatic determinations of osmium-fixed fat cells. *J. Lipid. Res.*, **12**, 521

6

The treatment of obesity by starvation and semi-starvation

A. N. Howard

COMPLETE STARVATION

Metabolic aspects

Complete starvation has been a subject of considerable interest to the academic scientist for many years[1], dating back at least to the classic experiments of Folin and Denis in 1915. The experimental work up to 1950 was extensive enough to justify a two-volume treatise[2], and the subject still forms a major interest in research on the 'dietary' control of obesity.

In modern developed society there is an abundant supply of food, but in the early history of man this was not always the case. The metabolic and psychological changes seen in complete starvation are the result of evolutional development essential to secure man's survival in periods of complete food deprivation. The chief need was to conserve energy and body metabolites essential for the continuation of life until food became plentiful. The source of energy is the adipose tissues which supply fatty acids and glycerol; only the latter is convertible to carbohydrate. The fatty acids are unable to be completely metabolized and end up as ketones. Probably the most important adaptation is that the brain switches over to using ketones as fuel rather than carbohydrate. The net effect of this is to conserve protein, which otherwise would necessarily have to be converted to carbohydrate.

The excretion of nitrogen drops dramatically and blood urea falls to low levels, indicating that little protein is being utilized for energy. Cahill[3] has calculated the origins and quantities of fuel consumed in man fasted for 5–6 weeks. About 150 g of adipose tissue and 20 g of protein is broken down in 24 h according to the scheme shown in Figure 1. Although the body can withstand prolonged periods of starvation, there are certain critical nutrients which are likely to be depleted first. Among these are potassium, sodium and vitamins such as C, B_1 and B_2.

139

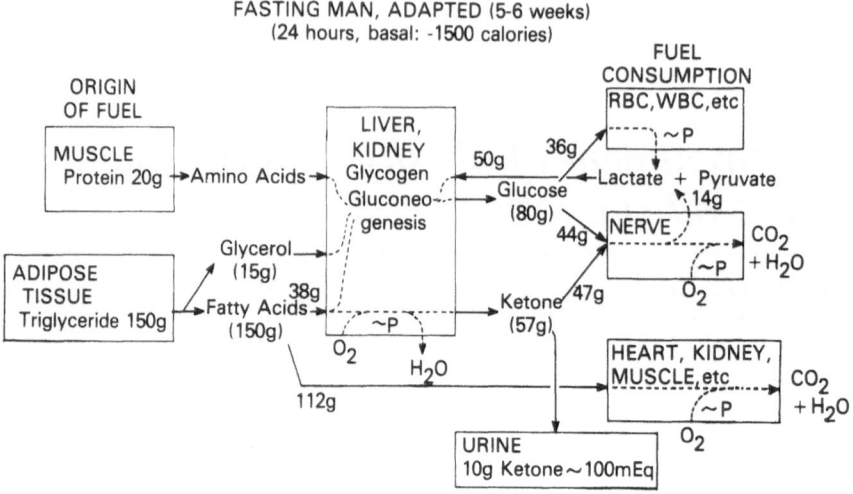

Figure 1   General scheme of fuel metabolism after 5 or 6 weeks starvation (from Ref. 3).

Frank deficiency of protein, iron and trace elements such as iodine will not appear until much later. Thus the major disabilities of complete starvation can be counteracted by giving adequate supplements of these vitamins and minerals.

Clinical effects of fasting

The so-called 'zero calorie diet' achieved great popularity in the treatment of gross obesity a few years ago and is still advocated with enthusiasm in certain parts of Germany[4]. Ideally the patient is required to spend periods of several months in hospital, although shorter periods of up to 4 weeks have been effective in selected outpatients. The regime consists of no food at all, water *ad libitum* but supplements of certain minerals and vitamins are prescribed as separate capsules[5]. A typical daily supplement consists of a multi-vitamin preparation containing iron (12 mg), and capsules of potassium (50 mEquiv) and sodium (40 mEquiv). Whilst it might be imagined that the patient would find this strict regime difficult because of intense hunger, this is not the case after the first 2–3 days because anorexia develops, and there is no compulsion to eat. Presumably this is a compensatory mechanism which has evolved as a psychological protection against long periods of food deprivation. The cause of the anorexia is unknown. The suggestions that the level of serum ketones which result from the catabolism of fat may inhibit the appetite centre is purely speculative[6].

Small quantities of carbohydrate (15–50 g per day), whilst suppressing the hyperketonaemia of starvation, do not increase hunger[7]. However, it is quite clear that, once food intake or volume is diminished below a certain level, anorexia develops.

An encouraging feature of the first week of treatment is the excellent weight loss of 4–7 kg, which is a great psychological stimulus to the patient. Only about half this is body fat, the rest being reduced volume of gastro-intestinal contents, and body water due to diuresis. In subsequent weeks the weight loss is about 3–4 kg per week, which diminishes the longer the patient is being treated.

The patient's mood and attitude is variable, mostly euphoric and garrulous but occasionally aggressive or depressed. It has been suggested that serum ketones have a pharmacological effect not dissimilar to alcohol, and that patients exhibit all the psychological symptoms of the alcohol drinker[8]. The euphoria seen in the first week of starvation is a large contributory factor in the success of 'health farms' since the client feels well, and also believes the excellent weight loss is chiefly body fat.

Starvation produces a rapid fall in basal metabolic rate of 20% or greater[9]. This is principally due to a fall in serum T_3 since the conversion of T_4 to T_3 is side-tracked so that an inactive isomer reverse (R) T_3 is chiefly formed[10]. In consequence, a mild hypothyroidism develops, and the patient will often complain of feeling cold, lethargic and may sleep more than usual.

Precaution

It is important to monitor the usual routine laboratory parameters frequently, and at least fortnightly. Decreases in serum total protein, albumin, haematocrit, haemoglobin and RBC occur because of protein lack. Of special importance are the serum electrolytes, since complete starvation causes an excessive loss of potassium, sodium and calcium. Dietary carbohydrate plays an important role in the retention of body electrolytes and the loss may be greater than normal. Appropriate additional dietary supplements of minerals are prescribed when and if necessary. Provided a multi-vitamin tablet is given as mentioned previously, no other deficiencies are likely.

Another consequence of the carbohydrate lack and ketosis is an elevation of serum uric acid to pathological levels, such as to lead to attacks of gout in a few patients[11]. However, the hyperuricaemia can be normalized by giving a xanthine oxidase inhibitor such as allopurinol routinely[12].

Whether a very high level of serum ketosis *per se* is harmful in man is unknown but lactic acidosis leading to a fatality has been reported. There is a condition in sheep known as 'pregnancy ketosis' in which the animals become anorexic and can eventually die[13]. The chief pathological effect is a fatty liver, no doubt due to excessive mobilization of fatty acids from the adipose tissue and deposition of triglycerides in the liver. An analogous situation may arise in human starvation.

Two laboratory parameters which may rise during treatment are creatinine[1] and bilirubin[14]. The cause of the former abnormality is reduced creatinine clearance due to a lower glomerular filtration, whilst the mild bilirubinaemia may result from a decreased uptake of haem by the liver. Serum cholesterol and triglycerides are beneficially decreased over the short term, but the former may rise to pre-treatment levels after several weeks[15].

During complete starvation, the excretion of urinary nitrogen is high during the first week but then plateaus at about the 4th or 5th week to 3·6 g N/day in men and 4·2 g N/day in women[16]. Over a prolonged period it would not be unexpected if signs of protein deficiency were not in evidence; anaemia can develop and a haemoglobin of 8 g/de and RBC of $3·0 \times 10^6/mm^3$, and neutropenia has been reported.

Complications

Common complications of therapeutic fasting include surreptitious eating, nausea and postural hypotension. Various cardiac arrhythmias have occurred and nutritional deficiencies will occur unless the appropriate supplements are given. There may be slow demineralization of bone, and alopecia and arrest of hair growth are common. Muscle cramps and colicky abdominal pain may occur, and other complications include menstrual irregularity with or without anovulation, loss of libido and decreased spermatogenesis. Some complain of fatigue, depression or inability to concentrate. Several deaths have been reported during therapeutic fasting[1]. One especially disquieting death was attributed to severe depletion of myocardial tissue during the re-feeding phase in a 20-year-old girl following a 30-week fast to less than her ideal weight[17]. It follows that, to be justified, fasting must result in lasting weight loss greater than that achieved by more conventional regimes.

Follow-up results

A number of series have reported the follow-up results of starvation undertaken for less than 4 weeks at the time of initial referral to a Hospital Clinic. The results are disappointing[18]. For example one study compared a group of subjects who were fasted for 10 days with 31 similar obese patients treated without fasting[19]. After a mean period of 21 months there was no significant difference in the overall weight change of the 30 fasted subjects available for re-assessment, and that of those treated with diet alone. The results of short-duration fasting in patients with 'refractory obesity' is even more disappointing[20]. Within a mean follow-up period of only 14 months all but one of 25 subjects regained all the weight loss achieved during fasting.

It has been suggested that starvation down to a personally and socially acceptable size might improve the follow-up results by providing a greater psychological incentive to adhere to subsequent dietary restriction, producing a more radical change in 'body image' and correcting the metabolic consequences of obesity. The results of such studies are generally disappointing, and even after prolonged starvation, massive weight regain is common. Thus after a mean follow-up period of 28 months only 11 of 75 massively obese patients were known to have maintained their weight to within 10 kg of that achieved by fasting[21]. A further study with a mean follow-up period of 7·3 years has recently been reported[22]. 121 subjects from a group of 207 morbidly obese patients were available for follow-up. Only seven had failed to regain weight; indeed 50% of the subjects regained their original weight within 3 years and this occurred irrespective of age of onset of obesity, duration of fast or degree of weight loss. However, many subjects who regain weight may benefit either physically or psychologically from the temporary weight loss they achieve, by obtaining employment, getting married, becoming pregnant or undergoing elective surgery[21,22].

Conclusions

It is possible that the follow-up results could be improved by the additional use of an intensive and prolonged behavioural modification programme, or by selecting only those patients who are most likely to succeed. Unfortunately, no method exists so far for predicting success. Until it does, the use of hospital beds for the treatment of obesity by complete starvation is not only expensive but also grossly inefficient. It can only be justified, if at all, when there is a pressing need to achieve temporary weight loss.

SEMI-STARVATION REGIMES

Simple protein-sparing regimes

To achieve nitrogen balance in complete starvation, supplements of proteins such as egg albumin or casein can be given. The strongest advocate of the protein-supplemented fast has been Blackburn[23], who gave patients 100 g casein per day with some mineral supplements. Weight losses achieved were not dissimilar to those seen in complete starvation. In view of this success, the food technologist was not long in producing protein products for over-the-counter sale. Most of these were liquid, based on hydrolysates made largely from cowhide, collagen and gelatin, to which saccharin and artificial flavouring was added[24]. The proteins included in such diets were nutritionally of low biological quality, and did not contain an adequate balance of essential amino acids. In the United States the business reached a high volume and over 50 brand names were on the market. Not unexpectedly, several deaths ensued, and of these, ten were shown definitely to be linked to the 'liquid protein' diet. Electrocardiographic information was available on seven, and of these five showed prolonged QT intervals and four of these five had low voltage. Serum potassium on admission ranged from 2·1 μEquiv/l to 4·2 μEquiv/l. Serum calcium, phosphate and magnesium were normal. Eight women died in hospital of ventricular arrhythmias despite efforts at resuscitation, including DC countershock and pharmacologic and electrolyte therapy. Pathological examination showed normal coronary arteries but myocarditis, mononuclear cell infiltration of the myocardium, and degeneration of the myofibrils. The FDA recommended that 'persons on such diets be closely followed by physicians. Electrolytes, specifically sodium, potassium, calcium and phosphate, should be monitored and ECG abnormalities watched for.' Besides the poor quality of the proteins used, the main problem with these liquid protein diets is the inadequacy of supplementary minerals and vitamins.

Supplemented protein-sparing regimes

There are a number of regimes in which supplements of vitamins and minerals are added. One very successful formulation, developed by Genuth et al.[25,26] used egg albumin as a protein of high biological value and carbohydrate as sucrose was included to give a composition shown in Table 1. Some minerals were present in the mixture, and supplementary vitamin tablets were given. However this formulation still remained low in calcium, phosphorus, magnesium, iodine and potassium. Although there is no recommended dietary allowance (RDA) for potassium, the conventional level included in most diets is 50 mmoles, whereas only 20 mmoles were prescribed.

Procedure

Genuth and his colleagues brought their patients into hospital for 7 days to institute the fast, during which time antihypertensive medication, diuretics, oral hypoglycaemic agents and insulin were withdrawn. Other drugs were generally continued. The diet was provided in sachets and given five times daily between 8 a.m. and 11 p.m.

Group sessions were held for the purpose of nutritional education, exercise training and family orientation. Following treatment in hospital, the patients remained on the same regimen, were discharged to follow their normal activities and seen weekly. The regime is terminated at or just above ideal weight. Every effort was made to transfer patients to a maintenance programme where various combinations of dietary regimes,

Table 1 Composition of supplement used in protein sparing modified fast[26]

Composition of Supplement	Daily intake	Percentage* RDA
Egg albumin	45 g	—
Glucose	30 g	—
Calcium	0·6 g	75
Phosphorus	0·35 g	40
Iron	18 mg	100
Magnesium	150 mg	40
Sodium	920 mg	—
Copper	tr.	—
Zinc	tr.	—
Manganese	4 mg	—
Essential fatty acids	2 g	100
Iodine	140 μg	0
Additional capsules		
Potassium (as chloride)	0·8 g	(40)
Vitamins (except E)	—	100
Energy content		
	320 kcal (1·34 MJ)	

* *Recommended daily dietary allowance.* Food and Nutrition Board, National Academy of Sciences. (Revised 1968)

augmented by individual and group therapy and intermittent supplemented fasting, were used as weight maintenance.

Results of treatment
In a study of 1200 patients, average starting weight was 106 kg for women and 136 kg for men. Seventy-five to 80% lost at least 18 kg (25–30% body weight). In successful patients (greater than 18 kg weight loss) the average total weight loss was 38 kg, equivalent to an average rate of 1·4 kg/week for women and 2·0 kg/week for men.

Improvement in diabetes mellitus, carbohydrate intolerance and hyperinsulinism were noted. In 67% hypertensive patients diastolic blood pressure fell to less than 90 mmHg.

Side-effects
Common side-effects encountered included transient initial diarrhoea, fatigue, orthostatic dizziness (rarely to the point of syncope), cold intolerance, skin dryness, hair loss, muscle cramps, amenorrhoea, decrease in libido and euphoria. However, the symptoms rarely caused premature termination of supplemented fasting. Five patients developed unilateral peroneal nerve palsy at the conclusion of weight reduction. Four recovered

promptly without specific therapy; one with prior sensory complaints in the distribution of this nerve required a brace for a year. Four patients with exceptionally large weight losses expressed a sense of confusion or disorientation with regard to their self-identity and body image and one required hospitalization for psychiatric treatment.

Four sudden deaths occurred (in 1200) in 4 years. One was accidental, the others all exhibited prior clinical and/or electrocardiographic evidence of heart disease, consisting of angina, ischaemic T-wave changes, remote myocardial infarction or multifocal premature ventricular contractions.

The chief biochemical abnormality was a slight elevation of serum uric acid stabilizing to 6–9 mg%. In a few patients where uric acid persistently exceeded 10 mg%, allopurinol or probenecid was found effective. No studies of nitrogen excretion under metabolic ward conditions were carried out. Hair loss, brittle nails, a tendency to low-grade anaemia (Hct < 33 in women and < 38 in men) and occasionally a decrease in visible musculature or complaint of muscle weakness were the only clinical manifestation of a possible loss of body protein. Serum albumin and transferrin levels remained normal.

Follow-up results

Of 47 patients who experienced successful weight reduction, and were examined about 22 months later, 55% had regained more than half the original weight loss and only 9% had maintained their body weight to within 10% of the original weight loss. Virtually all subjects who had regained substantially, expressed the desire to undergo a second course of treatment. However, in 63 patients who had regained more than half their original weight loss in the subsequent 5–40 months, a repeat course of supplemented fasting resulted in complete loss of regained weight in only 15 patients (24%). This compared with a success rate of 80% on a first course.

It is clear that the follow-up of patients is at least as important as the period of weight reduction itself. Two methods have subsequently been employed. In one group of patients, conventional dietary instruction was augmented by 1 week of supplemented fasting at regular intervals of 4–8 weeks, irrespective of the patients' weight.

In a second group, the total estimated needs of the patient were divided into a 'fixed' portion of highly regimented meal plans (70%) and a free portion which could be ingested as desired by the patient. The 'fixed' calories were hopefully interpreted as the same as the supplement with which they were treated initially. In addition, 1-week intervals of supplemented fasting were employed on an *ad lib* basis whenever the patient's body weight exceeded a designated upper limit.

Preliminary results covering a period of 15 months follow-up were mixed, and a trend towards failure was noted in each group. Certain individuals did extremely well but some 62/72 and 53/62 patients respectively in the two groups regained at least 50% of the weight lost. The percentage weight gain was less in those patients who attended a weight-maintenance clinic regularly. However, after treatment only 30% were motivated sufficiently strongly to continue attending a follow-up clinic. The possible reason given for this was that some patients exhibit resistance to continued contact with the nutritionist and physician. In others, there may be an unrealistic self-appraisal of their ability to manage on their own. Also embarrassment and guilt on gaining weight may make it difficult for the patient to re-attend. Whatever the reasons, the maintenance of weight loss remains a major problem in this type of therapy as it does for those undergoing complete starvation.

Very low-calorie conventional diets

The use of protein-based diets is not new. In contrast to the accepted teaching at that time, Evans, Strang and McClugage[27-29] published a series of papers between 1929 and 1931 claiming that a low-calorie diet of 400–600 kcal (1·68–2·52 MJ) could be used safely for the treatment of obesity. The diet went through a series of transitions. The earliest, Evans and Strang (1929)[27] consisted of the following daily: 2 eggs, 1 oz. bread, 3 oz. lean meat, 4 oz. vegetables and 1 cup bouillon. It contained 550 kcal (2·31 MJ), 26 g carbohydrate, 50 g protein and 27 g fat. This diet was deficient in potassium, calcium, magnesium, phosphorus, vitamins D, B_1, B_2 and nicotinic acid, according to current USA recommended levels. Later on, Strang *et al.* (1930)[28] replaced the eggs by egg-white and gave supplements of milk, orange juice and yeast. Viosterol as a source of vitamin D was added by Evans and Strang (1931)[29]. The complete composition of this modified diet is given in Table 2. It contains 400 kcal (1·68 MJ), 23 g carbohydrate and 50 g protein. Despite the various supplementations, the diet is deficient in potassium, calcium, magnesium, iron, phosphorus and vitamin A. Since recommended daily allowances had not been proposed at that time because of inadequate information, the incompleteness of the diet is not surprising. Although few routine laboratory tests were performed, an extensive series of experiments showed that the patients were in nitrogen equilibrium[29].

Patients were maintained on the diet at home without complications for 6 months and longer. In 295 patients studied between 1929 and 1936, the average period of dieting was 8 weeks[30], the average loss 9·9 kg or 1·2 kg per week, per person. In view of such good results it is strange that this particular diet should have been forgotten. Perhaps the reason is that it was rather monotonous and needed careful measurement of several ingredients to ensure success.

Table 2 Very low-calorie diet developed by Strang, McClugage and Evans in 1930[28]

MENU
10 oz. egg white (26 g protein)
1 oz. bread
3 oz. steak (beef)
4 oz. low calorie vegetables
50 c.c. whole milk
50 c.c. orange juice
50 c.c. yeast
salt
viosterol

COMPOSITION OF MAJOR NUTRIENTS

kcal (MJ)	403 (1·8)
Protein	50 g
Carbohydrate	23 g
Fat	12 g

CONTENTS OF MINERALS AND VITAMINS

	Daily intake (mg)	RDA*
Potassium	1235	60†
Calcium	204	25
Magnesium	93	25
Iron	6	33
Phosphorus	450	36
Vitamin A	2000 i.u. ‡	40
D	400 i.u.	100
B_1	2·1	200
B_2	1·7	170
Nicotinic acid	27	200
C	70	130

* *Recommended daily dietary allowance.* Food and Nutrition Board, National Academy of Sciences. (Revised 1968).
† Assuming requirement = 50 mEquiv/day
‡ Assuming vegetables were carrots (12 mg carotene per 100 g)

More recently the Simeons diet[31] has been extensively used by many medical practitioners, in conjunction with injections of human chorionic gonadotropin (HCG). Although the latter were shown to have the same effect on weight loss as saline, patients were strongly motivated to continue for 5–6 weeks, during which time the weight loss was 9–14 kg.

The diet is simpler than that described by Strang *et al.*, and is shown in Table 3. However, it does not contain the RDA of calcium, magnesium, iron and vitamin D. Over the relatively short period in which the diet is

Table 3   Nutrient content of Simeons diet[31]

Ingredient	g per day
Meat/fish	400
Green vegetables	200
Crispbread	30
Fruit	200
Energy content	500 kcal (2·1 MJ)

Nutrient	Estimated content (mg)	Percentage RDA*
Calcium	230	28
Magnesium	120	33
Iron	6	33
Vitamin A	1·0	130
B₁	2·7	250
B₂	3·0	200
C	60	110
D	0	0

* *Recommended daily dietary allowance.* Food and Nutrition Board, National Academy of Sciences. (Resised 1968)

used, these deficiencies would not be a serious consequence, but the diet is not recommended for longer than 6 weeks without appropriate supplementation.

Very low-calorie formula diets

Metabolic considerations
The fewer the calories a diet contains, the more difficult it is to include the recommended daily allowance (RDA) of minerals and vitamins while using natural foodstuffs. Below 1000 kcal (4·2 MJ) it is virtually impossible if a wide range of menus is desired. For this reason a formula diet containing the appropriate RDA of vitamins and minerals has many attractions, particularly if it can be made to simulate food such as soups or fruity desserts (Table 4).

With this concept in view, an attempt was made to define the optimum minimum daily requirements of protein and carbohydrate, consistent with good health and relative freedom from side-effects. Initial experiments[7] carried out in hospitalized patients at the West Middlesex Hospital, London, used a 'perfect mixture' of amino acids, oligosaccharides (hydro-

Table 4 Composition of very low-calorie* diet (Howard et al.[33])

	g per day
Protein[d]	31
Carbohydrate[e]	44
Fat[f]	2
Vitamins	[a]
Minerals	[b]
Guar gum	1
Flavouring	[c]

[a] Vitamins (mg): A, 0·85; B_1, 1·4; B_2, 1·6; B_6, 2·04; B_{12}, 0·049; C, 80; D_2 0·017; E, 33·7; K, 0·068; D-biotin, 0·205; calcium D-pantothenate, 10·2; choline bitartrate, 157; folic acid, 0·102; inositol, 119; nicotinamide, 18
[b] Minerals (mg); sodium, 1500;.potassium, 2000; calcium, 800–1100; phosphorus, 800; magnesium, 350; manganese, 4; zinc, 17; copper, 2·6; iron, 13; iodine, 0·16
[c] Calorie-free synthetic flavours such as chicken, asparagus, tomato, banana, strawberry, raspberry, etc.
[d] Milk proteins contained in skimmed milk solids, and calcium caseinate
[e] Lactose and sucrose
[f] Safflower or corn oil
* Manufactured by Organon, Oss, Holland

lysed starch), and the RDA of essential fatty acids, vitamins and minerals included in the preparation. The main object was to investigate the quantities of nutrients needed to ensure nitrogen equilibrium, electrolyte balance, and normal laboratory parameters. Following 2 weeks starvation, patients were placed on a carbohydrate-free diet and the amino acid mixture added stepwise in amounts of 20, 30 and 40 g per day. It was found that equilibrium was obtained at about 30 g per day (Figure 2). Carbohydrate was then added in quantities of 15, 30, 45 and 80 g per day. With increasing amounts the amino acid requirement fell and reached a minimum of 15 g per day at a level of 30–45 g per day carbohydrate. There was no further effect with 80 g per day. Essentially the same results were obtained when egg albumin was used as the protein source[32]. Thus it was concluded that between 15 and 25 g per day of high biological value protein and 30–45 g per day carbohydrate were the optimum. Although these results appear to conflict with others, earlier evidence that suggested that 50 g protein per day was essential may have failed to take into consideration the protein-sparing effect of carbohydrate itself, and also the fact that it requires 5 or 6 weeks for full adaptation to starvation to take place (as shown in Figure 1). This is illustrated in Figure 3 in which patients were given a diet containing 31 g protein, chiefly as casein[33]. During the first few weeks there was appreciable nitrogen loss, amounting to 56 g, but by the sixth week equilibrium was achieved. Studies in complete

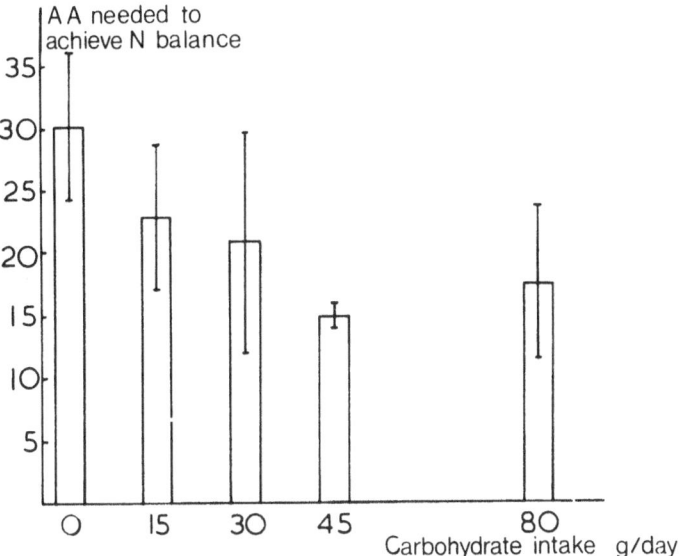

Figure 2 Effect of carbohydrate intake on quantity of amino acids (g per day) required to achieve nitrogen balance

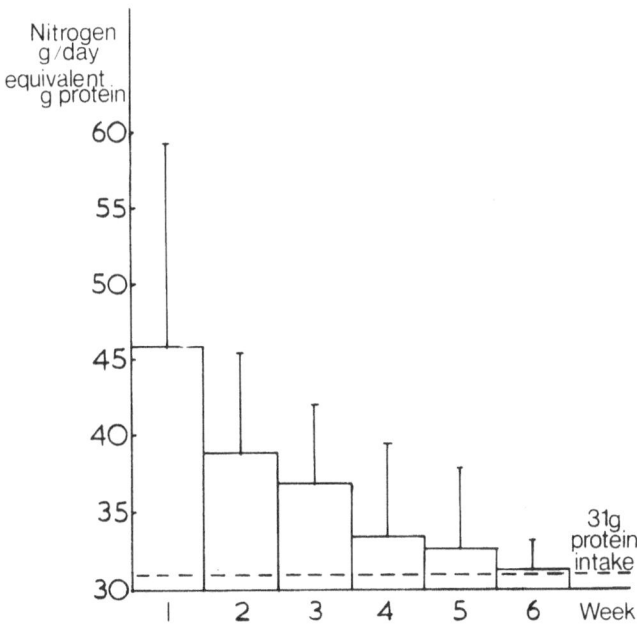

Figure 3 Nitrogen excretion in seven patients receiving 1·3 MJ per day formula diet containing 31 g per day protein

starvation[16] also indicate that after 4 weeks the nitrogen loss reaches a plateau equivalent to about 25 g protein. Thus these recent estimates of protein requirements are all consistent.

Although many investigators omit carbohydrate or reduce it to very low levels, the rationale for this is poorly based. The anorexic effects of fasting have been attributed to the high levels of serum ketones. However, the incorporation of as little as 15 g carbohydrate a day diminishes these metabolites and 80 g virtually abolishes them (Figure 4). These studies

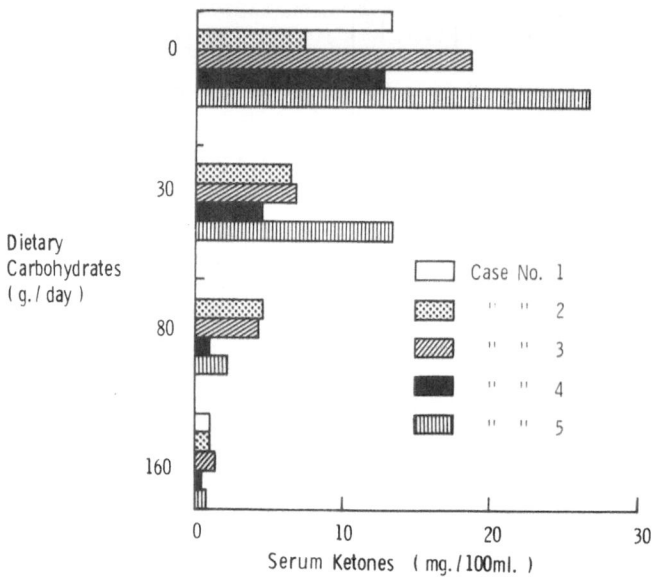

Figure 4   Serum ketone response to carbohydrate intake in five obese subjects

showed no correlation between serum ketones and hunger based on a linear rating scale. Thus, there is no important reason for admitting dietary carbohydrate which is an essential component of some important body constituents. In its complete absence protein has to be broken down, since the quantity of carbohydrate available from glycerol is inadequate (Figure 1). Excess of ketones is associated with increased uric acid production, and the latter also responds to dietary carbohydrate. A daily intake of 30–45 g of carbohydrate is sufficient to normalize the hyperuricaemia seen in complete starvation (Figure 5).

Electrolyte excretion and water retention is affected by carbohydrate intake. A zero-calorie diet leads to an excessive diuresis and loss of sodium and potassium in the urine[34]. Obese patients on high-carbohydrate diets of 1000 kcal (4·2 MJ) lose weight initially much more slowly than those on high-fat diets because of fluid-retention[35]. The phenomenon is also seen

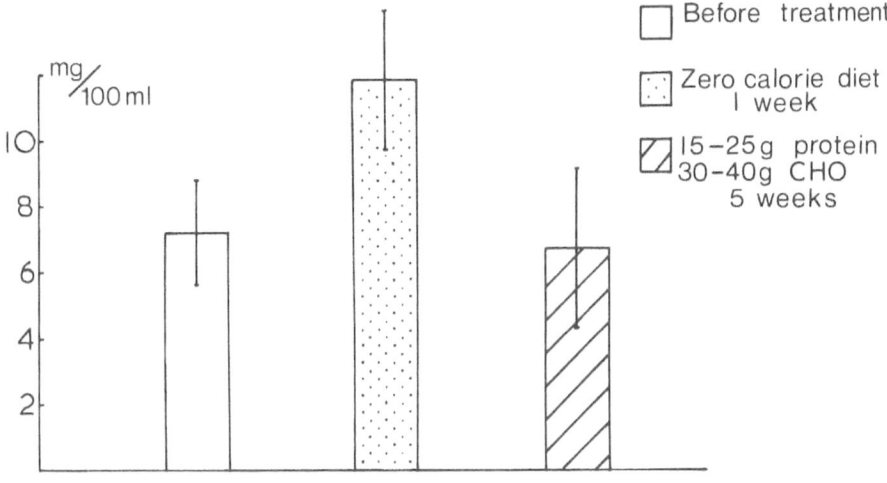

Group 1 and 2 combined

Figure 5   Comparison of the effect of starvation and very low-calorie diet on serum uric acid

with very low-calorie diets. Thus diets containing at least 80 g per day carbohydrate often lead to a slowing rate of weight loss and oedema. An optimum content is about 45 g per day, which is sufficient to prevent hyperuricaemia, ketosis and loss of electrolytes but insufficient to cause oedema.

In conclusion the ideal composition for a very low calorie diet is 15–25 g per day high biological value protein such as egg albumin and 45 g carbohydrate.

Side-effects

Using this regime the chief side-effects encountered in 52 patients were gastrointestinal. Four complained of occasional frequent loose motions attributed to insufficient fluid intake producing osmotic diarrhoea. In contrast five complained of constipation with mild to severe abdominal pain. This can be avoided by the addition of one small apple or 1 g guar gum per day to the formulation. Occasional thinning of the hair may occur, with spontaneous hair regrowth before recommencing a normal diet. Other side-effects, similar to those recorded by Genuth *et al.*[25,26] included dizziness, tiredness, feeling cold, and minor menstrual irregularities. Such complaints were transient, and were seldom reported more than once during the course of treatment. This contrasted with 12 patients who commented on a general feeling of well-being, an improvement to the growth of nails and texture of skin.

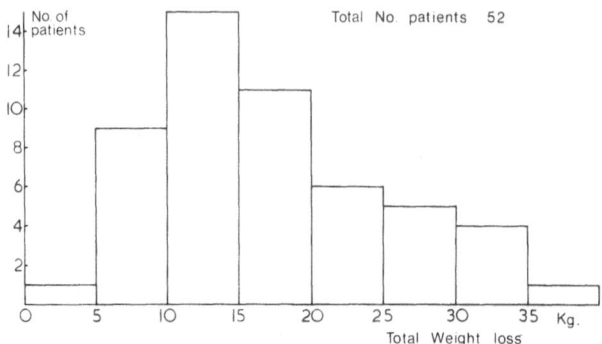

Figure 6   Distribution of weight losses in 52 patients treated with very low-calorie diet (180–320 kcal) containing egg albumin, for from 3 to 56 weeks

Efficacy

On such a regime the weight losses are highly satisfactory.

Figure 6 shows results on 52 patients who were admitted to hospital for 3 weeks, given an egg albumin diet and discharged as outpatients on the same diet for as long as they were able to continue. Of these studied, 77% were able to undergo a total treatment of 8 weeks and 54% for 16 weeks or over.

Seventeen patients came within 15 kg of their ideal body weight but at the end 67% could still be classified as obese (more than 20% above ideal weight). An example of a typical patient is shown in Figure 7.

Although studies on hospitalized patients are essential when metabolic parameters are being measured, it is impossible and too expensive to treat every obese patient by an initial training period in hospital. The egg albumin diet was therefore tried in a group of 38 outpatients. Since it was speculated that many would find the initial hunger too severe to continue the diet, the use of an anorectic drug suggested itself as a means of assisting the patient to overcome the initial distress[36]. For this purpose mazindol was chosen, since it is highly effective in producing anorexia rapidly in most patients. The study involved two groups of patients treated double-blind with mazindol or placebo for 8 weeks with a cross-over of the drug at the fourth week. Contrary to expectations, 66% of a group were to adhere to the 260 kcal (1·09 MJ) diet without receiving mazindol. There was no statistical difference in the mean weight loss between placebo and mazindol. The initial period of hunger which lasts only a day or two was well tolerated, and there seems little point in using supplementary anorectic drugs. The total mean weight loss was 9·3 kg at week 4 and 13·7 kg at week 8.

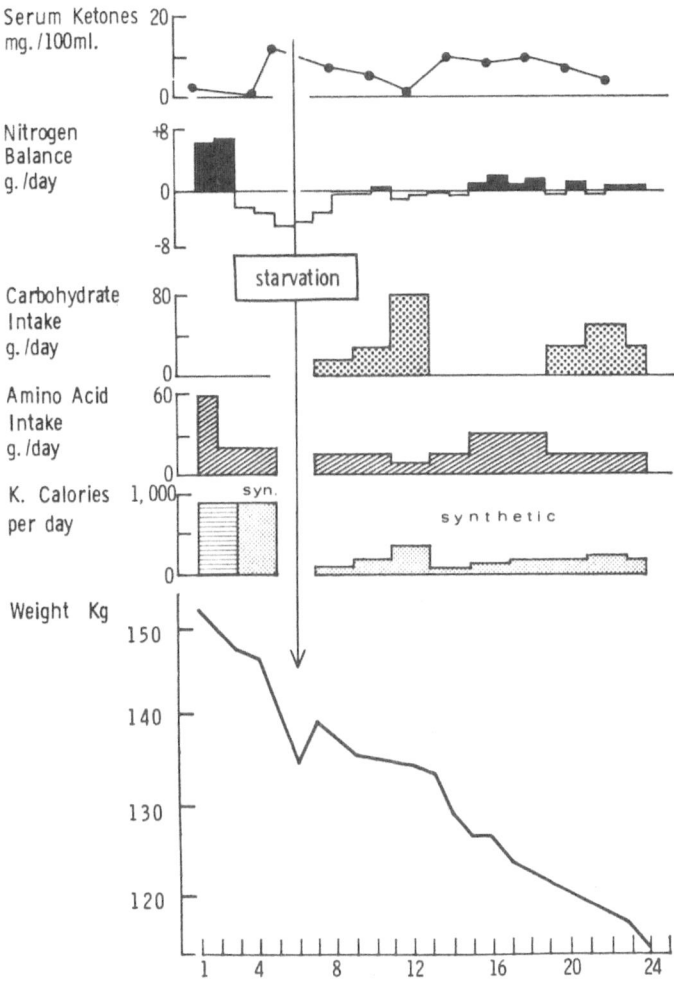

Figure 7 Effect of very low-calorie diet in a typical patient

In another study the weight losses of 22 hospitalized patients were compared with the same number of outpatients, this time using a 320 kcal (1·34 MJ) diet containing casein as the chief protein. As shown in Figure 8 the mean weight loss after 6 weeks was 2 kg greater in inpatients. However, after discharge there was no difference at the eighth week. Hospitalized patients find it more difficult to keep to a very low-calorie diet on discharge, presumably because they no longer have the security of the hospital to dissuade them from cheating. The general conclusion is that hospital treatment offers no major advantage for routine treatment and the additional expense is unwarranted.

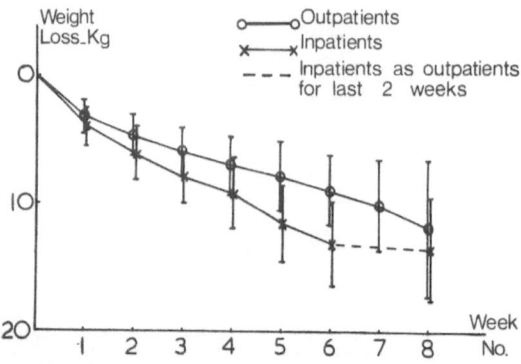

Figure 8   Mean weight losses ($\pm$ SD) in 22 outpatients and 7 inpatients on a
1·3 MJ per day formula diet

Palatability

One major problem remained: whilst the egg albumin diet was nutritionally ideal, its taste and texture were disliked without exception. Attempts
to flavour the formulation with tomato, chocolate, and fruit flavours in
order to produce something significantly more palatable, failed. The
texture of egg white is repellent to many patients, moreover it coagulates
on heating so the preparation of miscible hot drinks is impossible. Of the
proteins readily available probably the best alternative is casein, since it is
stable in hot water. Attempts to devise a formulation based on skimmed
milk products (Table 4) were highly successful, especially when the skills of
the food technologist were applied to the basic formulation. It is possible
to prepare various soups such as chicken, asparagus, and tomato, and
drinks and desserts such as chocolate, banana, raspberry and strawberry,
which are virtually indistinguishable from the usual household product and
can be enjoyed. Not surprisingly, the patient prefers a good-tasting diet to
one which can only be treated as a medicine. Whereas a dropout rate of
20% was usual with the egg albumin diet, because many patients found it
too unpalatable, a recent trial in 180 outpatients attending general practitioners gave a total of only five dropouts with the casein based formula.
One cannot ignore the organoleptic properties of formula diets. It is a
major factor in their eventual success.

PRACTICAL CONSIDERATIONS

The most efficient method of treating large numbers of obese patients by a
very low calorie regime either as conventional food or formula diet is to

hold a special weekly clinic. This has the great advantage that obese patients are able to meet outside the consulting room and discuss their treatment among themselves. It is helpful to have a discrete waiting area where up to ten patients can sit fairly close together. By not fixing a specified appointment time but allowing the patients to come between a fixed period of 2 hours (say 10 a.m. to 12 noon) patients are able to compare notes. It is often beneficial to start patients on the therapy in groups of up to ten with this purpose in mind. There will always be some who are more successful than others, and these leaders are a great stimulus to the rest, who can see the result of strict compliance.

In our Cambridge clinic, patients are referred by hospital consultants and general practitioners who give a brief idea of what is entailed in the treatment. Thus, only strongly motivated people and those without severe psychiatric disturbances are referred. At an initial interview a full explanation of the diet is given and the patients are asked if they are willing to try and complete a course of therapy lasting 12 weeks. Almost all will give a positive answer but a chance is given for the offer to be declined. Written instructions are given (see Appendix 1) with a supply of diet. Since most problems arise in the first week, it is beneficial to see the patient 1 week later and thence fortnightly.

At the beginning and every 8 weeks, RBC and haematocrit, electrolytes, creatinine, bilirubin, SGOT or SGPT and uric acid are measured. A weekly chart of objective impressions (Appendix 2) is filled in by the patient. This gives a chance to write down any particular problems which may arise, and guides the physician in prescribing auxiliary medication such as laxatives, hypnotics or anti-depressants, which may be deemed necessary. Appropriate forms for recording body weight, clinical and laboratory parameters, and medications are also of great value.

For research purposes it is often necessary to know if there is compliance or not. In complete starvation this is conveniently done by taking a sample of urine and using an aceto test strip for ketones, which should be positive. With very low-calorie diets containing carbohydrates this is impossible, since ketones are minimal or absent. A good method is for the patient to bring a complete 24 h specimen of urine and to have it analysed for sodium, potassium and urea. Since the electrolyte and nitrogen content of the diet is known, it is possible to estimate compliance. About 80–90% of the nitrogen intake is excreted as urea.

At the end of the specified period of, say, 12 weeks, the patient is re-assessed and a decision made as to whether a continuation is desirable or impossible because of lack of compliance. If the treatment is stopped the patient is offered a number of alternatives. These are; a conventional 600–800 kcal (2·52–3·36 MJ) diet; the very low-calorie diet during the working week and food at weekends; or the formula diet during the day and one low-calorie meal in the evening. Thus, by adopting the above procedures body weight can be maintained if the patient is seen monthly. Thereafter the patient may request the very low-calorie diet again after a 'rest' period of several months. However, a second attempt is rarely as successful as the first. Thus, it is best to encourage the patient to continue his initial attempt for as long as possible, at least until ideal body weight is reached.

A registrar and medical auxiliary can easily see ten patients per hour or even more. Thus, a typical weekly obesity clinic might have 30–40 patients in various stages of treatment at any one time. It is obviously important that patients should be discharged from the obesity clinic at a time when the long-term dietetic control has been standardized, otherwise it becomes impossible to take new patients.

FUTURE IMPROVEMENTS

A very low-calorie diet induces a mild hypothyroid state (Table 5), the BMR falls[37,38] by 20% and T_3 but not T_4 levels are decreased and RT_3 is unchanged in contrast to complete starvation, where it rises. These changes are seen as an adaptation process. The body is attempting to conserve energy and hence the rate of weight loss slows down.

Lethargy, fatigue, sleepiness and sensitive to cold are common complaints. It could be considered logical to give maintenance doses of T_3 (about 60 μg per day). This dose does not cause hyperthyroidism but produces normal, or slightly above normal, serum T_3 levels. An evaluation of this adjunct therapy is in progress, but the benefits, if any, appear difficult to assess since there is no spectacular difference between treated and untreated groups. Since thyroid medication increases nitrogen excretion[39], supplementation with T_3 presents a theoretical hazard in that tissue protein losses may be greater. Without further data on hospitalized patients, the magnitude of this effect is unknown, since previous investigators have employed much higher doses. The contraindications of T_3 are well known and should not be ignored.

Given that the patient complies, a consistent weekly and, with time, spectacular weight loss can be assured. Normal weight may eventually be achieved. However, this is only half the problem; follow-up is all-important. Only about 50% are permanently and successfully treated, the remainder increase their weight, usually to pre-treatment levels, within 1–2 years.

Further research is necessary to find out why there are so many permanent failures and what steps can be taken to achieve greater long-term success.

Table 5 Effect of 8 weeks treatment with a very low-calorie formula diet (320 kcal, 1·34 MJ) on BMR and thyroid hormones (Grant et al.[37])

	BMR (%)	Thyroxine (nmol/l)	Serum tri-iodothyronine (nmol/l)	Reverse T_3 (nmol/l)
Before start of diet	121 ± 13*	124 ± 23	1·7 ± 0·4	0·37 ± 0·18
8 weeks after start of diet	102 ± 8	117 ± 25	1·6 ± 0·3	0·4 ± 0·14
12 weeks after start of diet	99 ± 8	—	1·4 ± 0·3	—
Normal range	100 ± 14	55 – 144	1·0 – 2·8	0·14 – 0·53
P value at 12 weeks	< 0·01	NS	< 0·02	NS

* Standard deviation
NS = not significant

CONCLUSIONS

The treatment of resistant obesity by complete starvation can only be justified in exceptional circumstances if at all. Very low-calorie conventional diets offer a safer alternative, but it is impossible to include all essential vitamins and minerals in the food and supplementation with tablets or capsules are necessary. It follows that a complete palatable formula diet has many advantages, especially if given under medical supervision. It is preferable to the many variations of 'protein-sparing fasts' and 'liquid protein diets' which are invariably deficient either in carbohydrate or essential nutrients.

The outpatient treatment of resistant obesity can now be very successful in a high proportion of patients. However, the long-term outlook is still poor, and the chances of a complete 'cure' not greater than 50%. Further research is needed before the major problem of weight maintenance can be solved.

APPENDIX 1

Instructions given to patients given a very low-calorie formula diet

SPECIAL FORMULA DIET

The product you are given is a complete food. It contains all the essential nutrients to maintain you in good health. For success, *you must not consume any other food whatsoever*.

Instructions for use

Empty the packet into a large breakfast beaker (holding about 250 ml) and mix the powder into a smooth paste with a small quantity of cold water. Fill to the brim with hot or cold water as you prefer, mix well, and drink it immediately. If you are disappointed with its consistency a better mixture can be obtained using a food blender.

The diet is provided in several flavours. Take three sachets per day at mealtimes, corresponding to breakfast, lunch and dinner. It is important that you take all the diet – no more and no less.

Drinks

You are requested to drink plenty of fluids and, in addition to water, can take any of the following:–

(a) Tea or coffee without sugar. Saccharin can be used.

(b) Dietetic low-calorie fruit squashes (see that the label says not more than 1 calorie/fluid oz. (or 1 calorie/25 ml)). Calorie-free mineral (fizzy) drinks, e.g. 'Diet-cola, Schweppes Slim Line drinks'. If you are in any doubt, consult your doctor.

Alcoholic beverages, pure fruit juices and any drinks containing sugar are strictly forbidden.

Useful hints

1. On the first 2 days of the diet you may feel hungry in the evening. Either do something to keep your mind occupied or go to bed early. After a few days you will not feel hungry at all. If you do eat, it will make you feel very hungry indeed. So keep to the diet.

2. Indulge in all normal activities, but do nothing unusually strenuous (e.g. digging the garden, moving furniture, etc.). You will not feel especially tired, but if you do, sit down and take a rest.

3. You may find that your bowels will be opened less frequently, since the diet contains only a little bulk. Do not take any laxatives, if you feel constipated, but ask your doctor for his advice.

4. It is important that you see your doctor regularly, as arranged, in order to collect new supplies of diet. If you find one of the flavours highly objectionable, tell your doctor and replace it with another flavour.

IMPORTANT
You must keep to the special diet and take no other food whatsoever – only then will you lose a lot of weight.
Make up each sachet fresh and drink within 10–15 min. Otherwise the diet deteriorates.
Contact your doctor immediately if you have any urgent problem or need special advice.

APPENDIX 2

PATIENT'S ASSESSMENT SCALE

Name:_____ Date:_____

Please answer each question below placing a cross in one of the ten boxes next to the question.

The boxes at opposite ends of the rows represent opposite answers, and the other boxes represent all grades of answer between the two extremes.

This form should be completed weekly on Thursdays and handed in at the clinic.

How hungry do you feel?

Not hungry at all   Extremely hungry

What is your mood?

Depressed   Elated

How well are you sleeping?

Very badly   Very well

How much energy do you have?

None   Full of energy

How badly do you want to lose weight?

Not at all   Very much

Do you feel hot or cold?

Very hot   Very cold

How acceptable do you find the diet you are on?

Not acceptable at all   Extremely acceptable

What is your opinion of the flavour of the diet?

Disgusting   Excellent

The flavours I am using are _____

_____

Have you any other comments? _____

_____

References

1 Howard, A. N. (1975). Dietary treatment of obesity. In T. Silverstone (ed.). *Obesity: its Pathogenesis and Management* p. 123 (Lancaster: MTP Press)

2 Keys, A., Brozek, J., Henschel, A., Mickelson, O. and Taylor, H. L. (1950). *The Biology of Complete Starvation*, Vols. I and II (Minneapolis)

3 Cahill, G. F. (Jr.) (1970). Starvation in man. *N. Engl. J. Med.*, **282,** 668

4 Wechsler, J. G., Schonborn, J., Jager, H. and Ditschuneit, H. (1978). Changes in protein metabolism during total starvation. *Int. J. Obes.*, **3,** 390

5 Munro, J. F. (1973). The management of obesity. *Br. J. Hosp. Med.*, **10**(1), 8

6 Duncan, G. C., Jenson, W. K., Fraser, R. L. and Cristofori, F. C. (1962). Correction and control of intractable obesity. *J. Am. Med. Assoc.*, **181,** 309

7 McLean Baird, I., Parsons, R. L. and Howard, A. N. (1974). Clinical and metabolic studies of chemically defined diets in the management of obesity. *Metabolism*, **23,** 645

8 Bloom, W. L. (1959). Fasting as an introduction to the treatment of obesity. *Metabolism*, **8,** 214

9 Bray, G. A. (1969). Effect of caloric restriction on energy expenditure in obese patients. *Lancet*, **ii,** 397

10 Spaulding, S. W., Chopra, I. J., Sherwin, R. S. and Lyall, S. S. (1976). Effect of caloric restriction and dietary composition on serum T_3 and reverse T_3 in man. *J. Clin. Endocrinol.*, **42,** 197

11 Drenick, E. J. (1967). Weight reduction with low calorie diets. *J. Am. Med. Assoc.*, **202,** 118

12 Schatanoff, J., Duncan, T. G. and Duncan, G. G. (1970). Effects of allopurinol on hyperuricemia secondary to fasting. *Metabolism*, **19,** 84

13 Deuel, H. (1951-7). *The Lipids*. (New York: Interscience)

14 Fekete, J. T. and Sopou, E. (1978). Hyperbilirubinemia of fasting in obesity. *Int. J. Obes.*, **3,** 477

15 Spahn, U., Plenert, W. and Pathenheiner, F. (1967). Treatment by fasting in juvenile obesity. I. Changes of bodyweight during reduced energy intake and absolute fasting. 2. Free fatty acids in serum during drastic restriction of energy and during total starvation. *Z.Kinderheilk.*, **100,** 160; **101,** 20

16 Runcie, J. and Hilditch, T. E. (1974). Energy provision, tissue utilization and weight loss in prolonged starvation. *Br. Med. J.*, **2,** 352

17 Garnettes Barnard, D. L., Ford, J., Goodbody, R. A. and Woodhouse, M. A. (1969). Gross fragmentation of cardiac myofibrils after therapeutic starvation for obesity. *Lancet*, **i,** 914

18 Hoffman, R. (1978). Starvation diets in the treatment of obesity. *Obesity/ Bariatric Med.*, **7,** 10

19 Maagoe, H. and Mogensen, E. F. (1970). The effect of treatment on obesity. A follow up investigation of a material treated with complete starvation. *Danish Med. Bull.*, **17,** 206

20 MacCuish, A. C., Munro, J. F. and Duncan, L. J. P. (1968). Follow up study of refractory obesity treated by fasting. *Br. Med. J.*, **13,** 191

21 Innes, J. A., Campbell, I. W., Campbell, C. J., Needle, A. L. and Munro, J. F. (1974). Long term follow-up of therapeutic fasting. *Br. Med. J.*, **2,** 356

22 Drenick, E. J. and Johnson, D. (1978). Weight reduction by fasting and semi-starvation in morbid obesity. Long term follow-up. *Int. J. Obesity*, **2,** 123

23 Blackburn, G. L., Flatt, J. P., Cloves, G. H. A., O'Donnell, T. F. and Hensle, T. E. (1973). Protein sparing therapy during periods of starvation with sepsis or trauma. *Ann. Surg.*, **177,** 588

24 Editorial (1977). Details released at deaths of ten on liquid protein diets. *J. Am. Med. Assoc.*, **238,** 2680

25 Genuth, S. M., Castro, J. H. and Vertes, V. (1974). Weight reduction in obesity by outpatient semi-starvation. *J. Am. Med. Assoc.*, **230,** 987

26 Genuth, S. M., Vertes, V. and Hazelton, J. (1978). Supplemented fasting in the treatment of obesity. *Rec. Adv. Obes. Res.*, **2,** 370

27 Evans, F. A. and Strang, J. M. (1929). A departure from the usual methods of treating obesity. *Am. J. Med. Sci.*, **177,** 339

28 Strang, J. M., McClugage, H. B. and Evans, F. A. (1930). Further studies in the dietary correction of obesity. *Am. J. Med. Sci.*, **179,** 687

29 Strang, J. M., McClugage, H. B. and Evans, F. A. (1931). The nitrogen balance during dietary correction of obesity. *Am. J. Med. Sci.*, **181,** 336

30 Evans, F. A. (1938). Treatment of obesity with low calorie diets: report of 121 additional cases. *Int. Clin.*, **3,** 19

31 Simeons, A. T. W. (1954). The action of chorionic gonadotrophin in the obese. *Lancet*, **ii,** 946

32 Howard, A. N. and McLean Baird, I. (1977). A long-term evaluation of very low calorie semi-synthetic diets: an inpatient/outpatient study with egg albumin as the protein source. *Int. J. Obes.*, **1,** 63

33 Howard, A. N., Grant, A. Edwards, O., Littlewood, E. R. and McLean Baird, I. (1978). The treatment of obesity with a very low calorie liquid formula diet: an inpatient/outpatient comparison using skimmed milk protein as the chief protein source. *Int. J. Obes.*, **3,** 321

34 Bloom, W. L. and Mitchell, W. (1960). Salt excretion of fasting patients. *Arch. Intern. Med.*, **106,** 321

35 Pilkington, T. R. E., Gainsborough, H., Rosevoer, V. M. and Carey, M. (1960). Diet and weight-reduction in the obese. *Lancet*, **i,** 856

36 McLean Baird, I. and Howard, A. N. (1977). A double-blind trial of mazindol using a very low calorie formula diet. *Int. J. Obes.*, **1,** 271

37 Grant, A. M., Challand, G. S., Edwards, O. M., Wraight, E. R., Howard, A. N. and Mills, I. H. (1978). Thyroid hormone metabolism in obesity before and during semi-starvation. *Clin. Endocrinol.*, **9,** 227

38 Visser, T. J., Lamberts, S. W. J., Wilson, J. H. P., Doctor, R. and Henneman, G. (1978). Serum thyroid hormone concentrations during prolonged reduction of dietary intake. *Metabolism*, **27,** 405

39 Bray, G. A., Raben, M. S., Londono, J. and Gallagher, T. F. Jr. (1971). Effects of triiodothyronine, growth hormone and anabolic steroids on nitrogen excretion and oxygen consumption of obese patients. *J. Clin. Endocrinol.*, **33,** 293

7

Surgical techniques in the treatment of obesity

R. M. Baddeley

Ritual extremes of obesity practised by various races and countries, especially in Africa, have not generally been seen in Western Society. Even so, it has long been felt by the lay public that the fat person represents the ideal in happiness and contentment, even though physicians over 150 years ago cautioned that, in the extreme, obesity was a cause of early death.

It is now well known that with increasing weight the excess mortality above that of normal-sized persons rises alarmingly, to the extent that Life Assurance societies are reluctant to carry the additional risks. When a patient reaches 90% above standard body weight for age, height and sex, the excess mortality is 250% (16 times) greater than the norm[1]. The main causes of death are cardiac diseases, renal failure, accident and suicide, and even malignancy causes increased fatality. Increased morbidity due to hypertension, diabetes, orthopaedic disabilities, thrombo-embolism, gravitational ulceration, hiatus hernia, gall-stones and cirrhosis is common. Clinical diagnosis of unrelated conditions is more difficult as physical signs may be hidden by excessive adiposity. Surgical hazards are more likely as a result of technical difficulties and the higher incidence of wound and chest infections, deep vein thrombosis and pulmonary embolism. Social and economic handicaps abound due to family disharmony, inability to find or retain work and the additional cost of clothing.

Unfortunately, the results of conventional treatment have often been poor. Whilst it is relatively easy to induce weight reduction in the short term, it is much more difficult to sustain such reduction in the long term. Hence many patients spend their lives oscillating between greater and lesser degrees of obesity, never reaching grotesque proportions but rarely being slim. However, a few patients reach massive proportions, and in such people dieting is only rarely effective, not only because of the prolonged period of restraint required but also because of the lack of motivation. In such subjects, more radical and aggressive measures may be indicated, and during the past 20 years surgical methods have become increasingly employed.

The surgical procedures available to treat massive obesity are based on concepts of local removal of fat, induced hypophagia and malabsorption or prevention of hyperphagia. They include:

1. panniculectomy;
2. small bowel bypass;
3. gastric bypass;
4. dental splintage.

PANNICULECTOMY

The removal of excessive folds of fat from the abdomen (apronectomy), arms, thighs and breasts, has been practised for many years as a cosmetic procedure. This procedure does not influence the underlying problem of obesity and probably removes only a small percentage of excess weight. However, it may be psychologically beneficial in improving the patient's perception of body image and thus is an adjunct to other successful methods of weight reduction.

In one respect, apronectomy is physically beneficial. The presence of a large heavy abdominal apron tends to carry the centre of gravity to the body forward, causing straightening of the natural lordosis and ultimately backache. Removal of the apron of fat may restore spinal curvature and relieve backache.

SMALL BOWEL BYPASS

The use of iatrogenic malabsorption as a means of obtaining weight reduction was first recorded by Kremen, Linner and Nelson[2] in 1954. Two years later Payne and DeWind commenced their pioneering clinical studies, using the technique of jejunocolostomy. In this operation the jejunum was divided 37·5 cm from the duodenal–jejunal flexure and anastomosed end-to-side to the mid transverse colon to achieve malabsorption mainly of fat and to a lesser extent of carbohydrate and protein. In 1963 they reported their experience in 11 patients[3], and it was clear that metabolic hazards made this procedure unjustifiable.

The procedure was modified to retain the ileo-caecal valve and a small amount of ileum in continuity. This reduced the severity of diarrhoea by slowing somewhat the passage of bowel contents, preserving the full length of colon for fluid reabsorption and allowing some absorption of bile salts.

In 1969 they reported their experience in 70 patients using this less radical technique[4]. They found that optimal weight reduction was achieved by anastomosing the proximal 35 cm of jejunum end-to-side to the terminal 10 cm of ileum, retaining the defunctioned small bowel *in situ* to allow restoration of normal continuity should this become necessary due to untoward complications.

Since that time more than 2500 cases of jejuno-ileal bypass have been reported[5]. Various modifications to the surgical technique have been advocated and considerable experience obtained in the selection of patients and the incidence and management of side-effects.

Criteria of selection of patients for jejuno-ileal bypass

There is common agreement that surgical treatment is the last resort in the management of massive obesity and, as such, patients must meet the following stringent criteria before acceptance for investigations with a view to jejuno-ileal bypass:

(a) Chronic simple obesity of at least 5 years duration which has proved
(b) refractory to properly supervized dietary measures and is
(c) at least 45 kg or 100% above the standard weight for age, height and sex.
(d) The radical and aggressive nature of the procedure, its mortality and potential side-effects must be fully understood.
(e) There must be agreement to attend regularly for follow-up assessment as instructed by the clinician and to accept the advice given.

It is helpful to a patient to talk to other patients who have had the operation before a decision is made.

Pre-operative investigations

The pre-operative haematological, biochemical, radiological and other investigations routinely performed are listed in Table 1. Their purpose is to confirm the non-endocrine nature of the obesity and provide baselines for later comparison. To the list, percutaneous needle biopsy of the liver may be added if there is any abnormality in the biochemical liver function tests. A full psychiatric assessment is desirable, particularly in patients exhibiting overt psychiatric abnormalities.

Surgical procedures

The patient is prepared as for any small bowel procedure and the anaesthesia is similarly conventional. Prophylactic low-dose heparin and antibiotic are often prescribed, but matched blood for transfusion is not necessary.

The preferred incision is a midline mid-abdominal one skirting the

Table 1   Routine pre-operative investigations

Haematology
   FBC, Indices, ESR
   Folate, B_{12}
   Prothrombin time

Serum biochemistry
   Sodium, Potassium, Urea
   Calcium, Magnesium
   Creatinine, Uric acid
   Albumin, Globulin
   Bilirubin
   SGOT, Alkaline phosphatase
   Iron, Iron-binding capacity
   Cholesterol
   Triglycerides
   Cortisol
   T_4, T_3 uptake
Glucose tolerance
Total-body potassium
Skull X-Ray, ECG

---

umbilicus rather than a muscle-cutting one, because of the high risk of incisional hernia. The abdominal wall is retracted by a large strong self-retaining instrument in which the blades have been deepened to 12·5 cm. No other specially designed instruments are required.

The liver is checked for any abnormality and a needle biopsy obtained. Other viscera are examined, especially the gall-bladder, in view of the raised incidence of gall-stones in obese patients. The jejunum is measured along its stretched antemesenteric border from the Ligament of Trietz to the site of proposed transection using a piece of black silk or tape of the desired length. The measurement is repeated two or three times to obtain consistency of length. A similar technique is employed in measuring the site for anastomosis in the terminal ileum later in the operation. A 'window' is created in the jejunal mesentery by dividing appropriate vessels. The jejunum is then transected and the distal cut end closed with two layers of catgut. It is then anchored to the mesentery or transverse mesocolon with silk sutures. The jejuno-ileal anastomosis is then carried out by end-to-side or end-to-end technique in two layers. With the latter technique the free (proximal) cut end of ileum is implanted end-to-side into the ascending or transverse colon. The mesenteric spaces are then closed to prevent internal herniation.

It is routine practice to remove the appendix when present, and occasionally ovarian cysts. Other abnormalities, such as gall-stones, perhaps should not be removed because of impaired access due to adiposity and the desirability of not prolonging the anaesthetic in these patients. For the latter reason requests to perform abdominal apronectomy (panniculectomy) should be refused. The cosmetic result is better when performed after weight reduction has ceased. The abdominal wound is closed with nylon to the linea alba, dexon to the fat and silk to the skin. A vacuum drain may sometimes be employed in the very fatty abdominal layer. In women, a Foley catheter is left in the bladder to aid nursing care.

Post-operative management

Conventional regimes – intravenous fluid and electrolyte infusions and nasogastric suction – are followed. With the return of bowel sounds severe diarrhoea inevitably occurs, usually by the third or fourth day, and can be adequately controlled with diphenoxylate (Lomotil) 5 mg four times a day. Occasionally this may be supplemented with codeine phosphate and even cholestyramine. However, undoubtedly the most frequent cause of persisting excessive diarrhoea is attempted satiation of thirst by drinking large quantities of fluid. Because of the short length of bowel in continuity this has a purgative effect and exacerbates the diarrhoea, which in turn makes the thirst more marked. Thus patients are restricted to 1500 ml orally spread over 24 h, with beneficial effect[6]. Because of potassium loss with diarrhoea all patients should be given an oral potassium supplement which is continued until stool frequency stabilizes at two or three times daily.

On leaving the hospital the patients are advised to take a diet high in protein, low in fat and restricted in carbohydrate providing about 1500 kcal (6·28 MJ) per day. This an endeavour to achieve as normal a protein-calorie balance as possible.

The patient should be seen at monthly intervals for about 3 months and gradually increasing intervals thereafter, not being discharged from follow-up unless the jejuno-ileal bypass has been taken down and referred back to the General Practitioner for dietary surveillance. It is also wise to arrange routine annual inpatient assessments for liver and bone biopsies and for whole body potassium estimation, in addition to those investigations performed before the operation. These may be required more frequently if untoward side-effects occur.

Lengths of jejunum and ileum used in jejuno-ileal bypass

The length of bowel retained in continuity determines the efficacy of jejuno-ileal bypass in achieving weight reduction. When too much is retained weight reduction will not occur. When too little, the benefits of weight loss will be jeopardized by metabolic and nutritional problems. Thus considerable effort has been made to establish the lengths of bowel which achieve optimal benefit with minimal hazard.

The early clinical studies of Payne and DeWind[7] indicated that 35 cm of jejunum and 10 cm of ileum met these demands, and their results have been confirmed subsequently by others. Inconsistent weight reduction caused some surgeons to vary the type of anastomosis and the lengths of bowel utilized[8-10]. Salmon[9] used 25 cm jejunum and 50 cm ileum, Schwartz, Varco and Buchwald[11] 40 cm jejunum and 4 cm ileum, Gazet et al.[12] 10 cm jejunum and 25 cm ileum, and Corso and Joseph[13] 30 cm jejunum and 25–30 cm ileum.

Scott[14] compared four groups of patients in which four different lengths of bowel were used. Group one were of the Payne and DeWind type (35 + 10 cm end-to-side); group two 30 cm jejunum and 30 cm ileum; group three 30 cm jejunum to 15 cm ileum and group four 30 cm to 20 cm respectively, the latter three groups all having end-to-end anastomoses. The groups three and four patients lost weight more rapidly and ultimately achieved better weight reduction than groups one and two. Group three patients with the shortest lengths of bowel in circuit suffered more diarrhoea and metabolic difficulties than the others and they concluded that their preference was for the 30 + 20 cm dimensions of jejunum and ileum.

Another study[6] compared the weight reduction achieved in four groups of patients having the end-to-side type of anastomosis. The various dimensions used were 35 cm jejunum and 10 cm ileum; 10 cm jejunum and 35 cm ileum; 30 cm jejunum and 15 cm ileum; 30 cm jejunum and 10 cm ileum. There was no significant difference between any of these groups after 2 and 3 years follow-up and the metabolic hazards were similar throughout.

At the other extreme total lengths of bowel 'in continuity' measuring 70 cm or more induce little or no weight reduction. When the total length retained is 63 cm it does not matter whether the jejunum or the ileum is the longer[15-17]. Total lengths of 50 cm lose significantly less than those of 47 cm[18,19].

Thus the optimal length of bowel in continuity probably lies between 45 and 50 cm. In view of the hazards of protein–calorie malnutrition, it is probably judicious to retain longer lengths of jejunum than of ileum, though the longer the latter the less the likelihood of bile salt catharsis and vitamin B_{12} deficiency. Thus the author's present preference is for by-passes of 30 cm jejunum and 20 cm ileum as recommended by Scott[14], but utilizing the end-to-side anastomosis.

Types of anastomoses
The most commonly used type of anastomosis has been the end-to-side jejuno-ileostomy advocated by Payne and DeWind. Some, however, have found considerable variation in the amounts of weight loss by patients

undergoing the same operation and attributed this to reflux of bowel contents into, and absorption of nutrients from, the excluded ileum. In 1971 Scott[8] and Salmon[9] separately adopted an end-to-end technique of jejuno-ileostomy, the excluded ileum being implanted into the ascending, transverse or sigmoid colon. Scott[14] susbequently reported better and more consistent weight loss with this end-to-end procedure. Others, however, have remained unconvinced that this technique is more effective[6, 20–24]. In the first report two groups of 25 patients were randomly assigned to end-to-side or end-to-end jejuno-ileostomies, the lengths of bowel used in each being 35 cm jejunum and 10 cm ileum. In Figure 1 it can be seen that the weight reduction achieved was almost identical in both groups, studied for 5 years. The tendency to mild weight regain in both was similar, as was the incidence of side-effects. Mersheimer[24] found

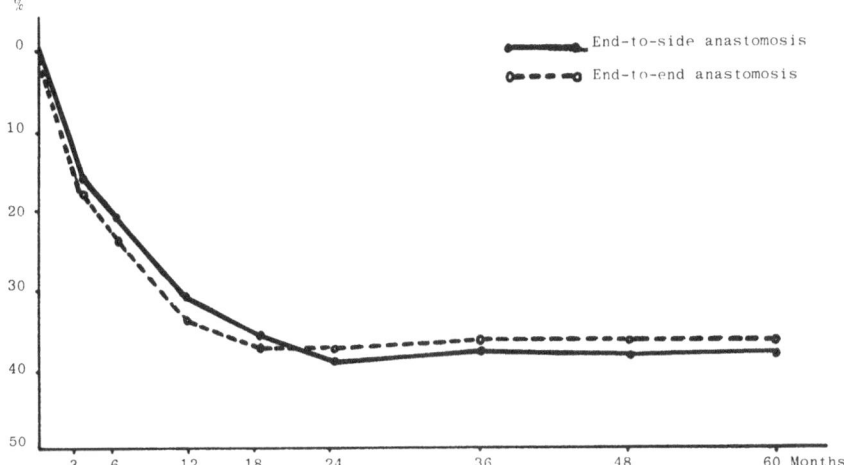

Figure 1 Mean percentage weight loss after end-to-side and end-to-end jejuno-ileal bypass

more frequent abdominal discomfort, diarrhoea, abdominal distension and bloating with the end-to-end type. In addition, recent reports of bypass enteritis and pneumatosis cystoides intestinalis (see later) have occurred in patients with this type of anastomosis where the ileum has been drained into the sigmoid colon.

The cause of weight reduction after jejuno-ileal bypass

It might be expected that the weight reduction achieved by jejuno-ileal bypass is due to malabsorption. However, following this operation food intake decreases considerably in all patients[5,16,22,25,26]. Bray[5] found that the pre-operative calorie intake in their group of patients averaged 28·1 MJ (6700 kcal) per day. During the first 6 months this spontaneously dropped to an average 5·53 MJ (1320 kcal) rising to 15·5 MJ (3700 kcal) per day by 1 year and nearly 21·1 MJ (5000 kcal) at 2 and 3 years. From this reduction in energy intake and estimates of energy expenditure it has been suggested that the weight loss achieved after bypass operations is due more to reduced dietary intake than to malabsorption[26].

It would thus appear logical to employ as long a bypass segment in continuity as is compatible with adequate weight loss, and to improve upon this by continuing the early spontaneous calorie reduction over the first 2 years of weight loss when the patient is most likely to respect the discipline of the surgeon in charge. The high protein-restricted calorie diet (approximately 1500 kcal (6·28 MJ) per day) should also reduce the frequency of diarrhoea and liver problems.

The beneficial effects of jejuno-ileal bypass

The main objective of jejuno-ileal bypass is weight reduction. This is dramatically and effectively achieved in the large majority of patients and is well sustained for many years. With it occurs reduction of blood pressure in about half of hypertensive patients[27, 28], correction of diabetes, decrease of serum cholesterol and triglyceride levels, improved respiratory function[29, 30], and notable psychosocial rehabilitation.

Pattern of weight reduction

Weight reduction occurs rapidly during the first year and usually amounts to about 30% of the original weight. Thereafter the process slows, so that at 24 months further reduction ceases. By this time the average loss has been 35–37%. Thereafter there is often a tendency to mild weight regain which may amount to as much as 10–12 kg. Most patients learn rapidly that this can be controlled by modest restraint of their food intake.

Table 2   Mean percentage weight loss after jejuno-ileostomy

Time	Mean percentage loss	Standard deviation	No. of patients
3 months	14·5	4·6	173
6 months	22·0	5·9	178
1 year	32·4	8·3	171
1·5 years	35·4	8·8	152
2 years	36·7	9·4	142
3 years	36·0	9·2	109
4 years	35·2	8·2	66
5 years	36·4	8·7	44

Table 2, however, shows large standard deviations implying that overall weight loss may be as little as 20% and as much as 50%. Thus whilst some may achieve close proximity to standard body weight others may remain far from it. If further weight loss is desired it is probably wise to utilize conventional dietary measures, or dieting enforced by dental splintage. Further bowel shortening increases the metabolic hazards while conversion to an alternative type of anastomosis often yields disappointing results. A better surgical alternative is to convert the jejuno-ileal bypass to a gastric bypass, as this would be easier in the slimmed patient.

The weight loss during the first year is predominantly fat, the loss of lean body mass being about half as much[31-33]. A somewhat different pattern was reported in one study[34] in which lean body mass declined during the first 3 months, levelled out and returned to pre-operative values by 1-2 years.

By two years, adaptive changes occur in the functioning jejunum and ileum which become dilated and elongated[35] and the mucosa becomes hyperplastic. Barry[36] found an increase of the crypt-to-villus ratio which implies increased production of epithelial cells. Functional changes in motility of the colon and of water and chloride shifts across the epithelium have been reported[37].

Psychosocial benefits

Patients with severe primary psychiatric disorders should not be selected for bypass because their post-operative behaviour and co-operation is unpredictable. Even so, it is to be expected that some personality disorder may be present if only because of the social limitation and humiliation of massive obesity. Many patients exhibit lack of self-esteem, strong fears of rejection, compulsions to please others, difficulties in self-assertion and distortion of body image[38]. Thus Abram[39] found that most patients exhibited mild passive aggressive, passive dependent and emotionally immature traits.

After operation the patients have usually exhibited mild euphoria as they look forward to being slimmer and healthier[40]. They become more physically and socially active and less self-conscious[39]. Their eating habits change to more normal patterns, and the tendency to compulsive gluttony disappears[41]. Even so, many act as though they are still large and the gradual reduction in body image takes place more slowly than the weight reduction itself[42].

There have been two reports[39,42] of significant psychiatric disturbance. Abram and colleagues[39] found that psychiatric difficulties occurred in 24% of thirty-four patients. Males and those with the greatest weight loss were most likely to be affected. The remainder, however, exhibited the very satisfactory benefits seen by other clinicians. The importance of careful selection is apparent.

As a consequence of psychological improvement the social benefits have been considerable. The restoration of normal ability to work either in the home or in employment has been of economic value. Some patients have obtained work for the first time in their lives. A few have even won beauty competitions!

Marital relationships have usually improved. Where marriage has irreversibly deteriorated, however, separation or divorce may occur as a result of greater confidence of the slimmed person to support him or herself and perhaps obtain another mate. Sometimes, improvement in confidence is retarded by embarrassment caused by excessive folds of redundant skin on the abdomen, arms and thighs. Such patients benefit from cosmetic surgery. Sexual performance probably differs little from that of the general population. Some exhibit loss of libido and others have prolonged amenorrhoea during the weight reduction phase[44]. The latter usually returns to normal spontaneously but the former may require testosterone implant therapy.

Pregnancy

There appears to be little hazard to pregnancy 2 years and more after bypass at which time weight reduction has ceased and intestinal adaptation has occurred[45]. Several authors have described lower birth weights than in previous pregnancies of their patients[46-50]. In conceptions occurring during the phase of rapid weight reduction, infant metabolic difficulties may arise due to maternal malabsorption and it is inadvisable for women to plan pregnancy at this stage.

Diabetes

A hazard of obesity is the development of diabetes, and it is well known that this can be reversed by weight reduction. Thus small bowel bypass may be expected so be similarly beneficial.

In a study of 13 patients who were either known diabetics or who were found to have diabetic glucose tolerance curves during routine pre-operative investigations, Fielding and Baddeley[51] found that all showed marked improvement when re-assessed 9–44 months later. Eight GTT had returned to normal, four were still mildly abnormal and one remained florid diabetic in type. All except one had achieved normal fasting blood glucose values and none required hypoglycaemic therapy.

The mechanism of this beneficial effect may be attributed to carbo-hydrate malabsorption[49,52], or increased insulin sensitivity evoked by weight reduction itself. Shibata[53] demonstrated impaired d-xylose absorption but found that this returned to normal 12 months after small bowel bypass. Others[16,54], found impaired d-xylose absorption for up to 18 months. During the early months, the glucose tolerance test yields a flat curve but with the restoration of normal d-xylose absorption it would be expected to resume a diabetic shape if the improvement were due to malabsorption. Furthermore, a patient who underwent small bowel reconstruction[51] did not re-develop her diabetes. Declines in plasma insulin levels[55] also occur, indicating a reduced demand during weight reduction. It thus seems that the beneficial effect on diabetes is related more to weight reduction and possibly increased insulin sensitivity than to carbohydrate malabsorption.

Serum lipids

The steatorrhoea which follows jejuno-ileal bypass is due to the shortness of the small gut and to partial interruption of the entero-hepatic circulation, a result of the reduced ileal surface available for cholesterol and bile salt absorption. The bile acid deficiency which occurs is compensated by increased synthesis in the liver[56, 57]. Serum cholesterol falls, and lipids are mobilized from peripheral stores to meet the demand.

There are dramatic falls of serum cholesterol values of 40–45% during the first 3 months after small bowel bypass[6, 14, 43]. This reduction is sustained for 5 years or more (Figure 2). Similar reductions occur in serum

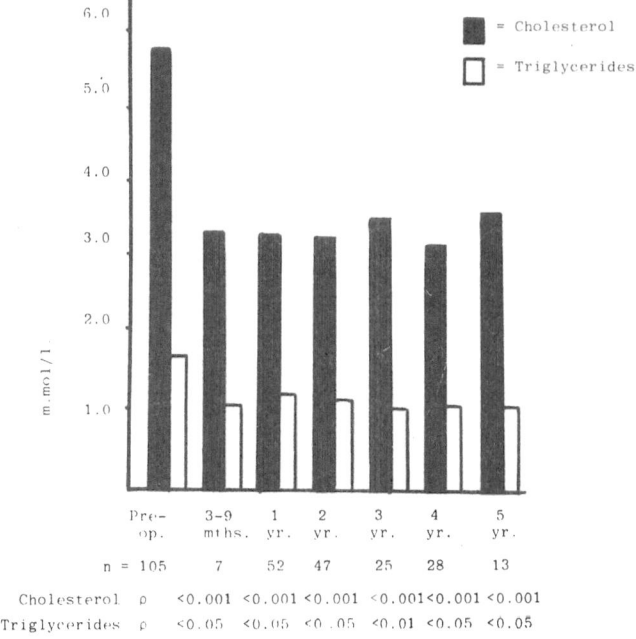

Figure 2 Changes in fasting serum cholesterol and triglycerides after jejuno-ileal bypass[6]

triglycerides, and type IV hyperlipoproteinaemic electrophoretic patterns have often returned to normal.

Mortality

The development of a new and radical surgical procedure like jejuno-ileal bypass will be associated with a relatively high initial mortality. The overall mortality culled from the world literature of some 2500 patients was 3·1%[5], ranging from 0 to 11·5%. Of these the operative mortality ranged from 0 to 6%.

The common cause of early death has been massive pulmonary embolism. Other causes include myocardial infarction, haemorrhagic pancreatitis, wound dehiscence, gram-negative septicaemia and inhalation of gastric contents. Outstanding as a cause of later death has been hepatic failure; less frequently myocardial infarction, pulmonary emolism, renal failure, gastrointestinal haemorrhage from oesophageal varices and intestinal obstruction due to adhesions or intussusception, have been responsible.

With greater experience and awareness, critical patient selection, and earlier effective treatment of side-effects, these mortality figures should be greatly reduced.

Morbidity

The main surgical difficulty in the post-operative period is fatty serous discharge arising from fat necrosis in the cut edges of the wound. Secondary infection frequently occurs and there is the ultimate hazard of wound dehiscence and incisional hernia. Deep vein thrombosis may be recurrent and require long-term anticoagulant therapy. Cases of hypoglycaemia and cirrhosis have been recorded[58] and deficiencies of fat-soluble vitamins A, E and K may occur. Serum carotene levels are always low in successful bypass patients. Patients may complain of their hair falling out; this is probably due to protein deficiency and usually ceases and is restored after a few months. The commonest complaint, however, is the cosmetic disability of redundant folds of skin and fat in the triceps region, the abdominal wall and the thighs, all of which may justify the appropriate panniculectomy.

The more significant complications of jejuno-ileal bypass listed in Table 3 are discussed in detail below.

Diarrhoea

This is not as severe a problem as might be expected. In the large majority the frequent watery diarrhoea of the early post-operative days and weeks settles steadily in response to oral fluid restriction and anti-diarrhoeal medication. Thus by 3 months the usual stool frequency is four or five times daily and after one year one to three times daily. During the first few months up to 25% of patients may experience excessive diarrhoea (more than six stools daily) causing anal soreness, exacerbation of haemorrhoids

Table 3 Complications of jejuno-ileal bypass

---

1. EARLY
    Wound infection
    Wound dehiscence
    Deep vein thrombosis
    Pulmonary embolism
    Incisional hernia
    Excessive diarrhoea

2. LATE
    Continued excessive diarrhoea
    Vomiting
    Fluid and electrolyte abnormalities
    Hair loss
    Fatty liver
    Cirrhosis
    Arthralgia and myalgia
    Renal and biliary colic
    Vitamin B_{12} deficiency
    Folate deficiency
    Abdominal bloating
    Foul flatus

---

and anal fissure. Marked thirst with polydypsia may occur. The thirst may be related to the fact that obese patients lose greater than normal amounts of fluid due to excessive sweating and insensible respiratory loss[31]. Rapid passage of consumed fluid through the shortened small bowel exacerbates the diarrhoea and evokes a vicious circle which may result in symptomatic fluid and electrolyte disturbance.

After the first year, diarrhoea is less troublesome though 80% of patients admit to occasional exacerbations after excessive or injudicious drinking and eating. It is rarely necessary to prolong anti-diarrhoeal medication beyond 6 months but some may need continuous treatment supplemented with cholestyramine.

Vomiting
Vomiting in the early weeks after operation may be due to electrolyte depletion or to actute fatty liver. It is usually controlled by metaclopramide but when persistent and severe may precipitate fluid and electrolyte depletion, especially when associated with excessive diarrhoea.

Fluid and electrolyte disturbance
Most reports of jejuno-ileal bypass surgery have indicated the hazard of fluid and electrolyte depletions. In the early months these are due to excessive diarrhoea, vomiting and, in some cases, hepatic failure.

Hypokalaemia causing marked weakness, muscle pain, cramps, nausea and further vomiting has occurred in as many as 25% of patients. Severe hypomagnesaemia is less common. It may present as carpopedal spasm, muscular twitches, irritability, anorexia, and ileus. Magnesium depletion may also cause retention of sodium and potassium within the bowel lumen, the cathartic effect of which provokes further diarrhoea[24]. Hypocalcaemia, occurs in 20–25% of patients in the early months, and when severe may also cause muscle cramps and carpopedal spasm[55,58,59]. A few patients also exhibit hyperchloraemic acidosis which may cause ataxia and inco-ordination[43].

In the author's experience of 230 patients, 200 of which have a minimum follow-up of 1 year, 32 have required hospital re-admission on one or more occasions. They were treated by saline and dextrose infusions containing potassium chloride, magnesium sulphate and calcium chloride. This regime effectively restored the wellbeing of those suffering purely fluid and electrolyte deficiencies. Thirst was reduced, enabling normal oral fluid intake and minimizing the problem of diarrhoea. Eighteen of these patients also had biochemical evidence of impaired liver function. After restoration of fluid and electrolyte balance, they were given amino acid infusion with benefit (see the section 'Acute fatty liver and liver failure', p. 181).

After 6–12 months, diarrhoea and vomiting become less troublesome and electrolyte disturbances infrequent. Whole-body potassium estimations, however, often give values in the lower normal range, and it is advisable to continue oral potassium supplements. Low serum levels become decreasingly frequent, occurring sometimes as a result of diarrhoea precipitated by dietary indiscretion, gastro-enteritis or antibiotic therapy for some other infective condition. In these circumstances patients are well advised to take extra potassium tablets without awaiting medical instruction.

Table 4   Incidence of low serum magnesium

Time (years)	No. of patients assessed	No. abnormal	Percentage incidence
0	181	1	0·6
0·25	158	28	17·7
0·5	158	29	18·4
1	156	33	21·2
1·5	144	18	12·5
2	133	33	24·8
3	110	34	30·9
4	63	24	38·1
5	36	15	41·7

Marginally low serum magnesium values have become increasingly frequent with time (Table 4). Usually this has been asymptomatic. When associated with low potassium values, oral repletion with magnesium gluconate or chloride, which have less marked cathartic effect than magnesium sulphate, is advisable as hypokalaemia may be less readily correctable in the presence of magnesium deficiency.

The subsequent development of calcium deficiency after jejuno-ileal bypass could be anticipated as a result of impairment of absorption. The reduced mineralization of bone recorded by Dano and Christiansen[60] was thus not unexpected. However, the absence of clinical evidence of skeletal deficiency seen by DeWind and Payne[43] who have the longest follow-up of any series, receives support from the author's personal experience. Low serum values after the first year are infrequent when correction is made for changes in serum albumin, and annual bone biopsies in 173 patients have not revealed a single case of overt osteomalacia after 5 years. The few late instances of hypocalcaemia have usually responded to oral supplement and vitamin D. Failure to respond to this treatment may be due to hypomagnesaemia[55].

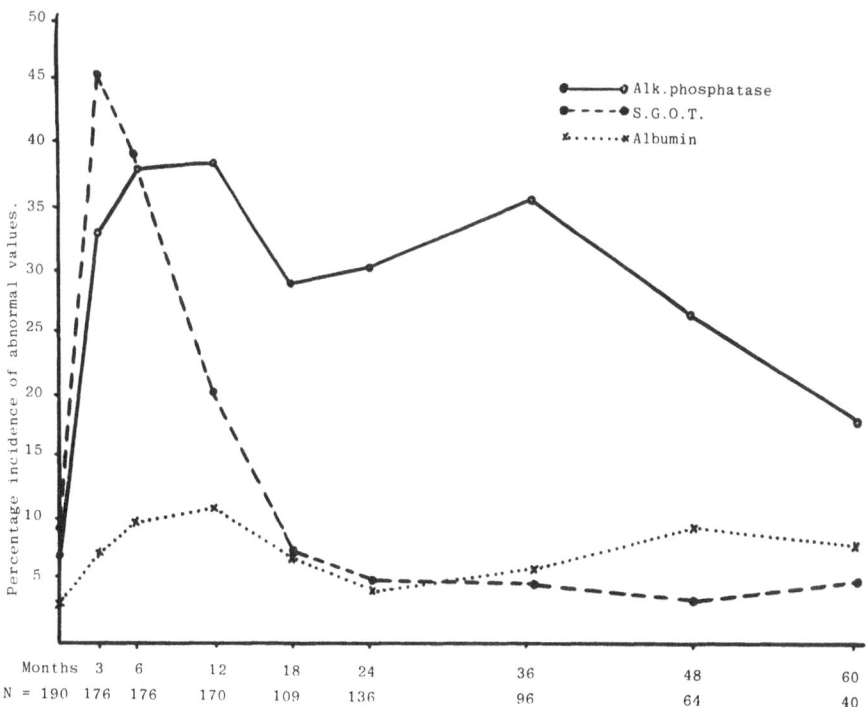

Figure 3 Incidence of abnormal liver function tests after jejuno-ileal bypass

Biochemical liver function tests
Routine biochemical liver function tests are often abnormal after small bowel bypass (Figure 3). The SGOT levels were abnormal in 46% of patients at 3 months but returned to the pre-operative incidence of abnormality after 18 months. Elevation of the alkaline phosphate may persist much longer. Likewise, sub-normal serum albumin levels, though less frequent, tend to continue. Most of these abnormalities were only marginal and were not associated with clinical evidence of hypoalbuminaemia.

These findings are in keeping with the observations of others[22,61,62].

Histological changes in the liver
The majority of massively obese patients have some degree of fatty infiltration of the hepatic parenchyma. The incidences range from 64% to 94%[6,15,16,63-66]. Males are more affected than females[63] and the heavier the patient, the greater the degree of abnormality[67].

Increase in fatty infiltration has been reported in all series during the first year following jejuno-ileal bypass. In the author's experience[6] (Table 5) this occurred in 55·4% of biopsies but tended to become less marked

Table 5 Changes in hepatic fatty infiltration after jejuno-ileal bypass

Year	No. of patients	Comparison with operative biopsy	
		No change/improved	Worse (percentage)
1	132	59	73 (55·3)
2	103	57	46 (44·7)
3	81	50	31 (38·3)
4	44	34	10 (22·7)
5	25	20	5 (20·0)

over the succeeding years. Even so, 5 years after surgery, 20% still exhibited increased fatty infiltration. Marubbio[66] showed that the distribution of fat was centrilobular or panlobular but not periportal, in the pre- and post-operative biopsies and the incidence of fatty change rose from 68% to 94% after 1 year. Much of the increase is due to triglyceride, present in twice the normal amount before surgery but rising 7 to 8-fold post-operatively[68].

The amount of fat present does not appear to correlate with various other changes that have been reported following operation. These changes include portal fibrosis and cirrhosis. The histocytic granulomata are of unknown significance; they contain multinucleate giant cells and have been seen in 28 of 175 biopsied patients, being present in four others in the original biopsy. The author[6] rejected four patients for surgery who were found to have early micro-nodular cirrhosis during their pre-operative assessment. Twelve patients (6·8%) post-operatively developed micro-nodular cirrhosis and two died in liver failure following restoration of small bowel continuity. This incidence is much higher than would be expected in UK patients and in only two could alcoholism be incriminated as an aetiological cause. The histological change was seen by one year in 6 patients, in the second year in 2, third year in 3 and fifth year in 1.

There have been several reports on the occurrence of cirrhosis after small bowel bypass[63,66,69-71]. Soyer[69] indicated that this change was reversible if the small bowel continuity was restored. The cause of concern is that these patients may be asymptomatic and biochemical liver function tests may be unhelpful. Unless routine liver biopsies are performed, the diagnosis may not be made until the cirrhosis is well advanced.

Acute fatty liver and liver failure

Although a large number of bypass patients exhibit biochemical and histological liver abnormalities, these changes are often asymptomatic and gradually improve spontaneously as weight reduction ceases. However, some show persisting abnormalities and may complain of lethargy, anorexia progressing to nausea and vomiting. A few become acutely ill; 18 of the author's series[6] of 190 patients showed symptoms of liver insufficiency confirmed by raised SGOT and alkaline phosphate, low serum albumin and rising bilirubin, and presaged the imminence of liver failure. Liver biopsies showed severe fatty changes. Vomiting may exacerbate hypo-kalaemia and hypomagnesaemia. This syndrome usually occurs in the first 6–12 months after the bypass and may prove fatal.

Symptomatic liver dysfunction demands immediate inpatient treatment for 10–14 days or more with intravenous concentrated amino acid infusions[72-74]. If the patient will take food, the diet should be high in protein and low in carbohydrate content. It is also probably wise to administer an antibiotic such as metronidazole to sterilize the bowel, which may be the source of hepatoxins produced by bacterial colonization. This regime will usually achieve a reduction in fatty change, improvement in liver function tests and restoration of the patient's state of well-being. However, failure to sustain the improvement demands repeated parenteral amino acids, and in such patients it is judicious to consider restoration of normal bowel continuity at an early stage.

Aetiology of liver changes after jejuno-ileal bypass

There are a number of possible explanations for these changes. They include protein–calorie malnutrition, excessive formation of lithocholic acid in the colon and its subsequent absorption, essential fatty acid deficiency and absorption of toxic bacterial products from the bypassed bowel.

There is good evidence of protein malnutrition after bypass[62,74] with impaired absorption and low serum values of many amino acids during the phase of marked weight loss. The reversal of fatty infiltration of the liver by intravenous administration of amino acid solutions[72] must suggest an aetiological relationship. White[75] likened the hepatic changes to those of kwashiorkor. This may not be strictly correct as bypass infiltration is primarily centrilobular, whereas in kwashiorkor it is periportal[76].

Because a small number of patients develop portal fibrosis and cirrhotic change with or without fatty infiltration, an additional toxic factor or factors may exist. The finding of high values of serum bile acids following bypass[77] suggested that this might be the hepatotoxic lithocholate fraction formed in the colon by bacterial action upon the large amount of unabsorbed chenodeoxycholate[78]. This theory has been discounted in humans as the problem does not occur after partial ileal bypass for hyperlipidaemia in which an even greater quantity of bile acids pass into the colon. Furthermore, one study has found no elevation of serum lithocholic acid in five patients who had post-bypass fatty infiltration[77]. There has also been no evidence in humans to support the malabsorption of essential fatty acids as the cause of the liver changes.

Similarities between the hepatic changes of alcoholism and those of bypass patients have been emphasized[79]. Only two of the author's twelve patients who exhibited cirrhotic change were alcoholic to any degree. The possibility that alcohols, formed by bacterial action in the colonized bypassed bowel, could be responsible for liver damage, has been discounted because they are not absorbed in sufficient quantities[80]. However, bowel colonization may well be responsible for the production of unidentified hepatotoxins. It is of interest that among patients undergoing restoration of small bowel continuity for a variety of side-effects those with severe hepatic dysfunction were colonized throughout with enteric organisms, whereas those with non-hepatic problems were not[6].

When the cause of liver abnormalities after small bowel bypass has been resolved, mortality and morbidity due to this complication should be greatly reduced and the main hazard of the operation minimized.

Bypass enteritis and pneumatosis intestinalis
In 1976 Passaro and colleagues[81] reported four patients upon whom end-to-end jejuno-ileostomy and ileo-sigmoidostomy, had been performed a few weeks beforehand, who experienced increased diarrhoea, fever, diffuse abdominal tenderness and distension. Straight X-ray of the abdomen revealed gaseous distension of the bypassed small bowel and fluid levels. Two patients underwent laparotomy which revealed oedema,

inflammation and dilatation of the excluded small bowel without obstruction, and pneumatosis cystoides intestinalis. They surmised that the condition was due to overgrowth of normal enteric flora and treated the last case satisfactorily with antibiotics.

Since then, a number of similar cases have been reported[82-84].

It is probable that enteritic symptoms such as those described by Passaro may also occur in patients with end-to-side jejuno-ileostomies, though so far, this complication has only been reported with the end-to-end ileo-sigmoidostomy type. It seems that the latter anastomosis is mechanically unsound because of the risk of sigmoid volvulus and because the motility pattern of the sigmoid may encourage reflux into the excluded ileum, thus promoting bacterial colonization. As there appears to be no significant advantage from this type of operation, the end-to-side technique should be the procedure of choice.

Polyarthralgia and polyarthritis

Migratory joint pains, often simulating rheumatoid disease, sometimes associated with polymyalgia, have been reported in up to 16% of patients in a number of series[43, 58, 85-88]. In the author's experience[6], 42% of 139 patients, followed up for 2 to 6 years, exhibited these symptoms to a variable extent. In most patients bouts last 1–4 days and settle spontaneously. In 11% they were severe and were sometimes prolonged. In two patients, severity and frequent relapse necessitated small bowel reconstruction with immediate and lasting relief. In none of these patients was pathological or radiological evidence of arthritic change seen, though such damage has been reported in other series. Serological tests for rheumatoid arthritis, antinuclear factor and LE cells have all been negative.

An analogy between this problem and the articular changes seen in inflammatory bowel disease has been drawn[88]. Evidence of circulating cryoprotein immune complexes and complement activation suggests systemic absorption of intestinal bacterial antigens, presumably from colonization of the defunctioned small bowel. The very good response in 48–72 h to courses of co-trimoxazole or metronidazole provides therapeutic support for this concept.

Renal and biliary calculi

The occurrence of oxalate stones and hyperoxaluria in jejuno-ileal bypass patients is comparable to that seen after major ileal resections for Crohn's disease, infarction and strangulation[89]. Dietary oxalate is normally bound to calcium in the gut and excreted in the stool. However, in the presence of steatorrhoea, calcium binds with the excess of fatty acids leaving free oxalate which is absorbed by simple diffusion. Being a metabolic end-product it is excreted in the urine and the absorbed excess may result in calculus formation.

The incidence of the problem ranges up to 30% in the several series reported[5], one of which recorded renal failure due to oxalate deposits in the kidneys[90]. Most surgeons have found 5–10% of patients have had one or more episodes of renal colic which occur at any time after the bypass operation.

Treatment by low oxalate diet has usually proved effective in reducing the likelihood of stone formation. Alternatively, or in addition, oral supplements of calcium or taurine, cholestyramine medication and low fat intake can be given.

The likelihood of increased incidence of biliary calculi after small bowel bypass has been less well substantiated as the problem has not been discussed in many of the reports of large series. Furthermore, obese patients are prone to gall-stone formation and a significant increase in the relative amount of cholesterol in bile has been recorded[91, 92] which may account for this incidence.

Even so, Wise and Stein[57] found 9·2% occurrence of biliary calculi in 65 patients after bypass and DeWind and Payne[43] 6·7% in 223 patients who were originally free of calculi. Mersheimer et al.[24] found new calculi in five of 44 patients.

Studies of bile composition have shown increased lithogenic index during the first 6 months, but thereafter this index returned to pre-operative levels[93]. The increased ratio of glycine to taurine conjugates in post-bypass bile[57, 94–96] may explain and support the contention of increased biliary calculi during the early post-operative months.

Abdominal bloating and foul flatus
Uncomfortable distension of the abdomen is a common complaint amongst bypass patients after the first year. It results from marked distension of the colon and is often associated with the passage of large quantities of foul flatus which provides temporary relief but is embarrassing. It tends to occur more towards the end of the day and most patients freely admit that it is more severe the more they eat[6].

The problem has been likened to megacolon[28] and intestinal pseudo-obstruction[97], there being no radiological evidence of organic obstruction and serum electrolytes remaining normal. Overgrowth of obligate anaerobic organisms are responsible for gas formation and the problem can be temporarily controlled by appropriate antibiotics such as metronidazole and tetracycline[93]. Unfortunately, resistant organisms may ultimately develop and so the first line of treatment should be dietary restriction to reduce the substrate available to bacteria, antibiotics being used when the response is inadequate. Occasionally the problem may be severe enough to cause the patient to request operation to restore small bowel continuity. Resection of dilated colon has proved ineffective and is not recommended.

Vitamin B_{12}, folate and iron absorption
Though part of the terminal ileum is retained in continuity in all jejuno-ileal bypass procedures, Schilling tests have shown impairment of vitamin B_{12} values in a number of series. Juhl and colleagues[98] found that serum vitamin B_{12} values gradually declined to subnormal levels over a period of 2 years in all ten patients they studied. Gastric acidity, intrinsic factor and serum vitamin B_{12} binding capacity values were normal and they considered that the short length of ileum and/or bacterial colonization of the proximal small bowel were responsible for the impaired absorption. As this could be improved with tetracycline therapy they incriminated the latter cause.

The importance of the length of ileum available for absorption was indicated in a study[95] which showed that vitamin B_{12} absorption was significantly less impaired if 36 cm of ileum were retained in continuity than if 12 cm were retained. The pattern of vitamin B_{12} malabsorption was different in patients with end-to-end compared with end-to-side anastomoses. In both types the Schilling test showed marked impairment immediately post-operation but with the end-to-end procedure improvement in absorption was seen at 6 months but not with the end-to-side patients. They presumed that the improvement in absorption was due to intestinal adaptation and that the failure to do so in the end-to-side group was due to bacterial colonization.

The long-term pattern of serum vitamin B_{12} changes are shown in Figure 4[6]. There was an increase in serum levels at 3 months followed by a steady fall. By 2 years, however, the large majority of patients showed steady levels lower than pre-operative values but well above the lower limit of normal. This steady state was maintained over the succeeding 3 years. In this series of 190 patients, three had low pre-operative values and seven subsequently required cyanocobalamin therapy.

Folate absorption normally takes place in the proximal small bowel and thus might be expected to remain normal after jejuno-ileal bypass. A large number of patients do, however, develop subnormal values, presumably due to bacterial colonization as normal serum levels can be rapidly restored by oral repletion therapy[6]. Thus there is need to monitor folate levels regularly to prevent the development of macrocytic anaemia.

Iron absorption occurs maximally in the proximal small bowel and may be expected to be unaffected by jejuno-ileal bypass. A number of reports have indicated the occurrence of iron deficiency but, as most of the patients undergoing this type of surgery are women, this is not necessarily

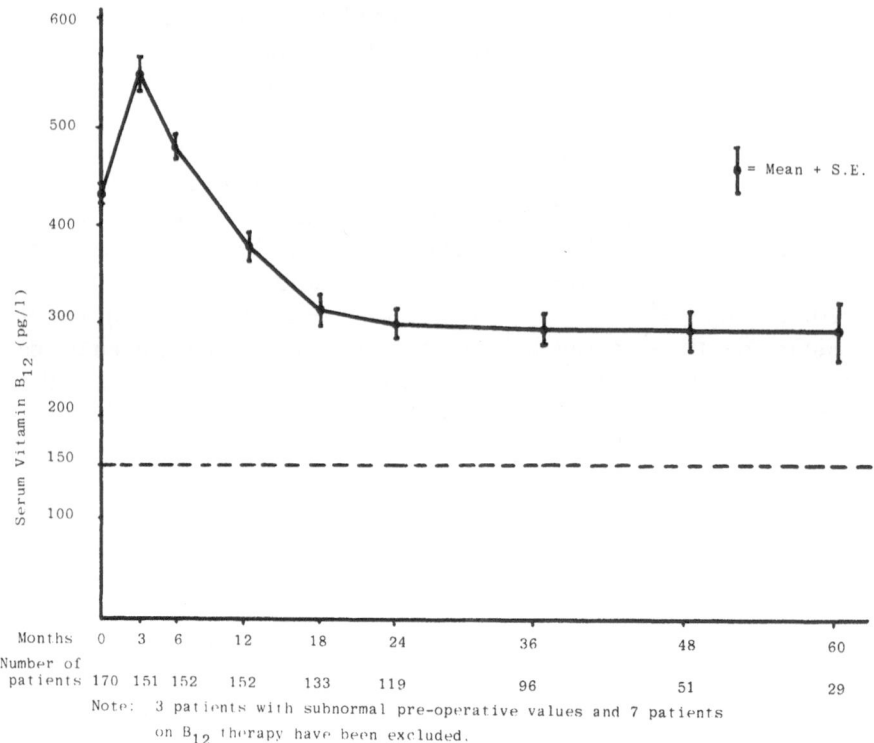

Figure 4 Serum vitamin B_{12} after jejunal bypass

attributable to the bypass. The incidence of iron deficiency in male patients was much lower[6].

Conclusions
Although jejuno-ileal bypass is an effective method of inducing and sustaining good weight reduction, its benefits are tempered by a large number of side-effects, some of which may be hazardous. On the other hand the large majority of patients are prepared to put up with these problems rather than the massive obesity with which they presented.

The weight loss will probably be improved by stringent dietary management, especially during the first 2 years. This would also reduce the potential liver hazards which constitute the main cause for concern during the first year. Mortality will be reduced by better awareness of the potentially lethal complications, by their early and aggressive treatment and by restoration of normal bowel continuity in those who do not sustain a satisfactory response to such treatment.

Refined patient-selection is imperative. Small bowel bypass should not be performed in patients of below average intelligence, as they seem less able to cope with the vicissitudes of the early months and often do not follow the instructions of their medical advisors. The Praade Willi syndrome is a strong contraindication to this operation as the hyperphagia they exhibit inevitably results in prolonged excessive diarrhoea which becomes a clinical and social problem. Severe primary psychiatric disability is unlikely to be improved by weight reduction and as the patients are unlikely to be reliable in their clinic attendances they too should be excluded. Alcoholism is also an obvious hazard.

Less strong contraindications are a history of heart disease, especially if recent in occurrence, as fatty change may also affect the myocardium. Perhaps patients over the age of 50 years should also be excluded, as they may lack the physical resilience required to cope with this operation and the difficulties of the early months. They are more likely to have myocardial ischaemia and pulmonary embolism.

GASTRIC BYPASS

Many years' experience of gastric surgery for peptic ulcer and cancer taught that extensive resections may cause loss of weight or, at least, failure to regain that already lost. Rapid satiety due to the small capacity of the gastric remnant (small stomach syndrome) and the discomfort evoked by food from dumping and vomiting, in effect reduced calorie intake to an adequate minimum. In 1965, Mason of Iowa, USA, applied a concept of the small stomach syndrome to the treatment of massive obesity and others have since followed his example having found that good weight reduction can be achieved without some of the side-effects seen after jejuno-ileal bypass[100-110].

Criteria for selection of cases for gastric bypass

The same criteria of case selection applied to jejuno-ileal bypass candidates are appropriate to those for gastric bypass. As there appear to be fewer nutritional side-effects it may be also suitable for lesser cases of gross refractory obesity and for those patients who have already slimmed successfully and are at risk of regain. The latter may include those previously treated by dental splintage enforced dieting, or cases of complicated jejuno-ileal bypass which have required reconstitution[107]. Gastric bypass has also been used in children and cases of Praade Willi syndrome[104] in which there is reluctance to use jejuno-ileal bypass.

Pre-operative assessment and preparation

This follows the same lines as those of jejuno-ileal bypass, but it is also helpful to have radiological assessment of the oesphagus, stomach and duodenum to exclude peptic ulceration or hiatus hernia.

It is common practice to employ low-dose heparin and antibiotic therapy for prophylaxis against deep vein thrombosis and sepsis. In all other respects patients are prepared in a manner applicable to any gastric procedure. Because of the hazard of splenic injury cross-matched blood should be available.

Operative technique and post-operative management

Mid-line upper abdominal incisions do not allow easy access in the massively obese for a procedure which even in slim patients may be difficult. Better access can be achieved by a supra-costal curved transverse incision[108] in which the rectus muscles are detached, drawn caudally and a transverse incision made in the peritoneum. The upper part of the stomach can then be mobilized, but it may be necessary to remove the spleen in so doing. A high transection is then performed to create a small proximal pouch of about 10% of the entire gastric volume. The use of a stapling

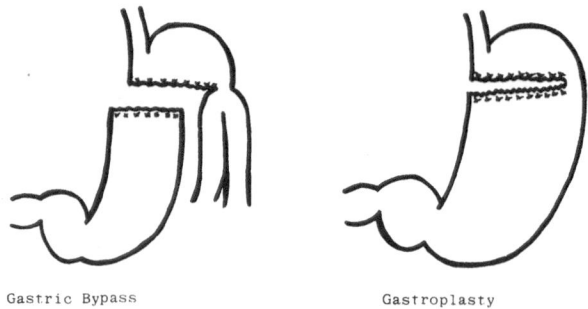

Gastric Bypass   Gastroplasty

Figure 5   Gastric surgery for obesity

device in this manoeuvre is expeditious. A loop of proximal jejunum, as short in length as possible, is then anastomosed retrocolic to the proximal pouch creating a stoma no larger than 12 mm diameter[110] (Figure 5). The importance of anchoring the stoma below the transverse colon has been emphasized, but because of difficulty in so doing, others[106] have used a Roux-en-y technique with jejuno-jejunostomy 30 cm distal to the gastro-jejunostomy. This has the added advantage of reducing the potential problem of bile vomiting. Antecolic gastro-jejunostomy has also been used[110]. The distal closed 90% remnant is usually anchored to the anterior surface of the proximal part to prevent torsion. Thus, like jejuno-ileal bypass, the procedure is reversible if later undesirable effects occur.

An alternative technique, gastroplasty[102] (Figure 5), in which the stomach is maintained in continuity but partially transected to leave a narrow passage between the proximal (10%) part of the stomach and the distal (90%) has been abandoned because of disappointing weight loss.

The post-operative management of gastric and intestinal ileus follows the traditional lines of intravenous infusion, nasogastric suction and gradually increasing quantities of clear fluid. By the fourth day small feeds may be tolerated, but nausea and vomiting can cause delay. On discharge the patients should be encouraged to take three soft meals daily, the importance of maintaining adequate protein and vitamin intake being emphasized.

Results of gastric bypass

The largest series of cases is that of Mason and colleagues[111] who, in 1975, reported their experience in 442 patients, 57 of whom underwent gastroplasty. Seventeen of the latter required conversion to gastric bypass because of poor weight loss. Forty gastric bypass patients required revision operations to narrow the stoma in order to improve weight loss. Three patients required discontinuance of the bypass and re-anastomosis of the proximal and distal gastric segments.

The operative mortality was 3% and overall mortality 5% (22 patients). Four patients died from pulmonary embolism, one from acute liver failure, nine from peritonitis, four from cardiac causes, three from cancer and one from progressive hepatitis known to be present prior to operation. More than a quarter of the deaths have occurred in patients over the age of 50 years.

Morbidity consisted mainly of wound sepsis, which is common in obese patients; vomiting, which may be due to over-eating and drinking; stenosis of the stoma and early cardiorespiratory difficulties, which may be related to the prolonged duration of the operation as well as the gross extent of the obesity. Dumping syndrome occurs in about one-third of patients and stomal ulcer in 1·6%. Late metabolic effects are, however, infrequent, though problems of osteomalacia may be anticipated after several years. The histological changes in the liver seen after jejuno-ileal bypass are less frequent.

Weight reduction varies from patient to patient but Mason found the average weight loss was 36 kg at 1, 2, 3 and 5 years post-operation. About one-third lost 50 kg. Similar weight reduction at the 1-year stage has been obtained in other series[109,110]. Older patients lose less weight than young adults[103] and mild regain of weight may occur in some after reduction has ceased. Gastric bypass in children under 20 years[104] achieved 15% weight loss at 6 months and 25% at 3 years. Cases of Praade Willi syndrome did less well.

Comparison of gastric and jejuno-ileal bypasses

There have been three clinical reports comparing the benefits and hazards of gastric and jejuno-ileal bypass[106,109,110].

Griffin and colleagues, in a randomized prospective study[106], found no significant difference in the weight loss achieved by both techniques after 1 year, but it should be noted that the length of the jejuno-ileal segment retained in continuity was 5 cm longer than that advocated by Payne and by Scott. Mortality was similar in both groups, but early complications were more frequent in the gastric bypass patients. The incidence of late surgical complications was low in the latter patients, consisting mainly of recurrent nausea and vomiting. In seven, bilious vomiting required conversion of the jejunal loop to a Roux-en-y reconstruction which even then was not always curative. Fatty infiltration of the liver tended to improve in most patients after gastric bypass.

In an unrandomized consecutive series[109], gastric bypass patients showed better weight reduction than the preceding jejuno-ileal bypass patients at 1 year with clinically excellent or good results in 83% of the former compared with 42% of the latter. In Alden's[110] unrandomized series, the results of 100 patients receiving a modified gastric bypass operation were compared with 100 earlier patients treated with a Payne type of jejuno-ileal bypass. Both groups achieved similar weight loss at the 1-year stage but there was less morbidity in the gastric bypass patients.

Conclusion

Gastric bypass results in fewer late complications than jejuno-ileal bypass. The latter is, however, technically easier to perform whereas the former is a particularly difficult and lengthy operation carrying greater risk of peritonitis, splenectomy and respiratory complications. Thus the operative mortality may be expected to be higher. It remains to be seen whether the weight reduction of gastric bypass is sustained in the long term and whether the side-effects of jejuno-ileal bypass necessitate increasing need to restore intestinal continuity. As inevitably the latter commonly results in regain of the weight loss, it may be worth considering conversion to gastric bypass, as this procedure would be much less difficult in the thinner patients[107].

The incidence of stomal ulcer after gastric bypass is low, varying from 1·6%[111,112] to 6%[105]. Dumping symptoms may require narrowing of the gastrojejunostomy stoma. Persistent vomiting may be due to bile reflux or stenosis of the stoma. Hence the need for revision operations may be higher than after jejuno-ileal bypass

The problem of cirrhosis after jejuno-ileal bypass which occurs in as many as 6·9% of patients[6] is a serious hazard which may require discontinuance of the shunt. After the first 12–18 months fatty liver becomes much less of a problem. It should be possible to minimize the hazard of hepatic insufficiency by insisting on a high-protein, low-carbohydrate diet. Late discomforts due to abdominal bloating and foul flatus appear to be the main cause for complaint in these patients, and in some who cannot control the problem by dietary restraint, reversal of the procedure may be requested.

Thus, both procedures have drawbacks which will be improved by refinements of technique, management and case-selection. Undoubtedly they both achieve great social and psychological benefits which probably occur earlier with gastric patients and are more variable with jejuno-ileal patients. Many years of follow-up must elapse before their roles in the management of massive obesity can be truly evaluated. In the meantime their use should be confined to those with a special understanding and interest in the subject of obesity and knowledge of the pathophysiological changes which may occur.

DIETING ENFORCED BY DENTAL SPLINTAGE

Conventional dietary techniques of weight reduction are often unsuccessful because of inability to adhere to the regimes imposed or to sustain the reduction once achieved.

Failure to adhere to diets may be due to mood changes which compel impulsive or episodic over-eating. This not only halts the weight reduction but often reverses it, thus evoking further depression and diet-breaking. Dental splintage prevents impulsive over-eating by physical restraint of mastication.

The selection of cases for dental splintage is similar to that of other surgical methods of obesity treatment. It is essential that the patient's dentition should be satisfactory and that the desired motivation should be present. Many patients prefer to undergo intestinal bypass despite its major radical nature as they clearly wish to continue eating. They are, thus, not ideally motivated and probably will not achieve a good result unless actively encouraged to continue the technique by frequent follow-up discussions.

The technique of interdental splintage and the dietary regimes employed have been described by Wood[113] and Rodgers[114]. The fluid diet used is based on milk or soup amounting to 800 kcal (3·35 MJ) with additional iron and vitamin supplements. The patients are usually weighed fortnightly or monthly. If weight reduction has not been achieved the large majority of patients can be accused of erring from the regime. The frequency of breakage of interdental wires may convey further indication of inadequate motivation. The dental caps are removed at 3-monthly intervals for purposes of hygiene, and replaced if necessary.

Both patients reported by Garrow[115] lost over 40 kg in a period of 5 months. Weight loss occurred in all 17 patients studied by Rodgers but three defaulted or were unwired within 1 month. Median rate of weight loss declined from 9 kg per month to 1·5 kg per month over 6 months, amounting to 25·3 kg in ten patients over 6 months.

In the author's experience of 53 patients, 42 completed 6 months treatment. Of the remainder six could not tolerate the restraint, two were managed elsewhere, one became pregnant and two failed to return to the clinic. Average weight loss was 4·15 kg per month and amounted to 25·8 $\pm$ 9·63 kg.

The side-effects of dental restraint enforced dieting are few and are easily managed. Occasional cases of hypoglycaemia, hair loss and depressive tendency have occurred but usually can be treated without discontinuance of the regime. Haematological and biochemical profiles have remained consistently satisfactory.

The technique has the obvious advantages of relative cheapness and minimal loss of time from work. A major disadvantage compared with intestinal or gastric bypass is the likelihood of weight regain after removal of the splints. This can only be minimized by stringent dietary re-education and vigilance at a clinic or by the general practitioner. It remains to be seen whether the short-term benefits are sustained for, if they are no better than those of other dietary methods, the dental and medical time and expense involved will not be justified in the context of the heavy demands made on the National Health Service.

GENERAL CONCLUSIONS

Surgical treatment is necessary only in the few patients who become massively obese and remain refractory to conventional dietary management. In these, dieting enforced by dental restraint is an effective, simple and relatively inexpensive regime which carries little risk. It is not applicable to those with inadequate dentition and is abhorrent to some, mainly women. It is imperative that re-education of eating habits is achieved after completion, otherwise regain of weight will inevitably occur.

Of the gastrointestinal procedure, gastric bypass is gaining in popularity as it has less morbidity than jejuno-ileal bypass yet appears, in the short term at least, to be equally effective in achieving weight reduction. It is, however, technically more difficult and thus may carry a higher operative mortality. In either case the importance of careful patient selection cannot be over-emphasized. It is recommended that its use should be confined to centres experienced in the subject, for only then can the potential hazards of such radical measures be minimized and a good standard of results achieved.

References

1 Jaggers, C. L. (1976). Personal communication
2 Kremen, A. J., Linner, J. H. and Nelson, C. H. (1954). Experimental evaluation of nutritional importance of proximal and distal small intestine. *Ann. Surg.*, **140**, 439
3 Payne, J. H., DeWind, L. T. and Commons, R. R. (1963). Metabolic observations on patients with jejunocolic shunts. *Arch. Surg.*, **106**, 432
4 Payne, J. H. and DeWind, L. T. (1969). Surgical treatment of obesity. *Am. J. Surg.*, **118**, 141
5 Bray, G. A., Greenway, F. L., Barry, R. E., Benfield, J. R., Fiser, R. L., Dahms, W. T., Atkinson, R. L. and Schwartz, A. A. (1977). Surgical treatment of obesity: a review of our experience and an analysis of published reports. *Int. J. Obesity*, **1**, 331
6 Baddeley, R. M. (1978). The management of gross refractory obesity by jejuno-ileal bypass. (Hunterial Lecture, Royal College of Surgeons of England, 24th February, Birmingham)
7 Payne, J. H. and DeWind, L. T. (1969). Surgical treatment of obesity. *Am. J. Surg.*, **118**, 141
8 Scott, H. W., Sandstead, H. H., Brill, A. B., Burk, O. H. and Younger, R. K. (1971). Experience with a new technique of intestinal bypass in the treatment of morbid obesity. *Ann. Surg.*, **174**, 560
9 Salmon, P. A. (1971). The result of small intestine bypass operations for the treatment of obesity. *Surg. Gynecol. Obstet.*, **132**, 965
10 Buchwald, H. and Varco, R. L. (1971). A bypass operation for obese hypolipidaemic patients. *Surgery*, **70**, 62
11 Schwartz, M. Z., Varco, R. L. and Buchwald, H. (1973). Pre-operative preparation, operative technique and post-operative care of patients undergoing jejuno-ileal bypass for massive exogenous obesity. *J. Surg. Res.*, **14**, 147
12 Gazet, J. C., Pilkington, T. R. E., Kalvey, R. S., Crisp, A. H. and Day, S. (1974). Treatment of gross obesity by jejuno-ileal bypass. *Br. Med. J.*, **4**, 311
13 Corso, P. J. and Joseph, W. L. (1974). Intestinal bypass in morbid obesity. *Surg. Gynecol. Obstet.*, **138**, 1
14 Scott, H. W., Dean, R. H., Shull, H. J., and Gluck, F. (1977). Results of jejuno-ileal bypass in two hundred patients with morbid obesity. *Surg. Gynecol. Obstet.*, **145**, 661.
15 Weismann, R. E. (1973). Surgical palliation of massive and severe obesity. *Am. J. Surg.*, **125**, 437
16 Bray, G. A. (1976). *The obese patient*, vol. 9. (Philadelphia: W. B. Saunders)
17 McLean, L. D. (1976). Intestinal operations for obesity; a review. *Canad. J. Surg.*, **19**, 387
18 Baden, H. (1974). Bypass operations in treatment of obesity. *Ann. Chir. Gy.*, **63**, 365
19 Quaade, F. (1977). Studies of operated and non-operated obese patients: an interim report on the Scandinavian obesity project. *Am. J. Clin. Nutr.*, **30**, 16
20 Quaade, F., Juhl, E., Feldt-Rasmussen, K. and Baden, H. (1971). Blind loop reflux in relation to weight loss in obese patients treated with jejuno-ileal anastomosis. *Scand. J. Gastroenterol.*, **6**, 537
21 Backman, L. (1975). Rate of weight loss after intestinal by-pass operations for obesity – analysis of factors of significance. *Acta. Chir. Scand.*, **141**, 424

22 Benfield, J. R., Greenway, F. L., Bray, G. A., Barry, R. E., Lechago, J., Mean, I. and Schedewie, H. (1976). Experience with jejuno-ileal bypass for obesity. *Surg. Gynecol. Obstet.*, **143,** 401

23 Gaspar, M. R., Movias, M. J., Rosental, J. J. and Anderson, D. (1976). Comparison of Payne and Scott operations for morbid obesity. *Ann. Surg.*, **184,** 507

24 Mersheimer, W. L., Kazarian, K. K., Dursi, J. F. (1977). A critical analysis of 51 patients with jejuno-ileal bypass. *Surg. Gynecol. Obstet.*, **145,** 847

25 Mills, M. J., and Stunkard, A. J. (1976). Behavioural changes following surgery for obesity. *Am. J. Psychiat.*, **133,** 527

26 Pilkington, R. R., Gazet, J. C., Ang, L., Kalucy, R. S., Crisp, A. H., and Day, S. (1976). Explanations for weight loss after ileo-jejunal bypass in gross obesity. *Br. Med. J.*, **1,** 1504

27 Iber, F. L., and Cooper, M. (1977). Jejuno-ileal bypass for the treatment of massive obesity. Prevalence, morbidity and short and long-term consequences. *Am. J. Clin. Nutr.*, **30,** 4

28 Fikri, E. and Casella, R. R. (1974). Obesity: jejuno-ileal bypass for obesity – results and complications in 52 patients. *Ann. Surg.*, **179,** 460

29 Jacobsen, E. M., Dano, P. and Skovsted, P. (1974). Respiratory function before and after weight loss following intestinal shunt operation for obesity. *Scand. J. Respir. Dis.*, **55,** 332

30 Soterakis, J., Glennon, J. A., Sihihara, A. M., Tyler, J. M. and Iber, F. L. (1976). Pulmonary function studies before and after jejuno-ileal bypass surgery. *Am. J. Dig. Dis.*, **21,** 553

31 Brill, A. B., Sandstead, H. H. and Price, R. (1972). Changes of body composition after jejuno-ileal bypass in morbidly obese patients. *Am. J. Surg.*, **123,** 49

32 Scott, H. W., Brill, A. B., and Price, R. R. (1975). Body composition in morbidly obese patients before and after jejuno-ileal bypass. *Ann. Surg.*, **182,** 395

33 Spanier, A. H., Kurtz, R. S., Shibata, H. R., MacLean, L. D. and Shizgal, H. M. (1976). Alterations in body composition following intestinal bypass for morbid obesity. *Surgery*, **80,** 171

34 Goldberger, J. H., Cha, C., Hazard, W. L. and Randall, H. T. (1976). Jejuno-ileal bypass for morbid obesity – early results and body composition changes in 45 patients. *Surgery*, **80,** 493

35 Fenyo, G., Backman, L. and Hallberg, D. (1976). Morphological changes of small intestine following jejuno-ileal shunt in obese subjects. *Acta. Chir. Scand.*, **142,** 154

36 Barry, R. E., Barisch, J., Bray, G. A., Sperling, M. A., Morin, R. J. and Benfield, J. (1977). Intestinal adaptation after jejuno-ileal bypass in man. *Am. J. Clin. Nutr.*, **30,** 32

37 Rask-Madsen, J., Bruusgaard, A., Munck, O., Nielsen, M. D. and Worning, H. (1974). The significance of bile acids and aldosterone for electrical hyperpolarisation of human rectum in obese patients treated with intestinal bypass operation. *Scand. J. Gastroenterol.*, **9,** 417

38 Solon, C., Silberfarb, P. M., and Swift, K. (1974). Psychological effects of intestinal bypass surgery for severe obesity. *N. Engl. J. Med.*, **290,** 300

39 Abram, H. S., Meixel, S. A., Webb, W. W. and Scott, H. W. (1976). Psychological adaptation to jejuno-ileal bypass for morbid obesity. *J. Nerv. Ment. Dis.*, **162,** 151

40 Castelnuovo-Tedesco, P. and Schiebel, D. (1976). Studies of super-obesity.

2. Psychiatric appraisal of jejuno-ileal bypass surgery. *Am. J. Psychiat.*, **133**, 26

41 Brewer, C., White, H. and Baddeley, R. M. (1974). Beneficial effects of jejuno-ileostomy on compulsive eating and associated psychiatric symptoms. *Br. Med. J.*, **4**, 314

42 Kalncy, R. S., Solow, C., Hartman, M. and Crisp, A. H. (1975). Self reports of estimated body widths in female obese subjects with major fat loss following ileo-jejunal bypass. In A. N. Howerd (ed.). *Recent Advances in Obesity Research* **1**, (London: Newman)

43 DeWind and Payne, J. H. (1976). Intestinal bypass surgery for morbid obesity. *J. Am. Med. Ass.*, **236**, 2298

44 Editorial (1978). Dietary amenorrhoea. *Br. Med. J.*, **1**, 321

45 Baddeley, R. M., and Fielding, J. W. L. (1977). Pregnancy after jejuno-ileal bypass, *Internat. J. Obesity*, **1**, 121

46 Everett, R. B., Crosby, W. M., Welch, J. D. and Thompson, J. B. (1974). Pregnancy after jejuno-ileal bypass for obesity. *Surg. Gynecol. Obstet.*, **139**, 215

47 Barron, J., Frane B. and Bozalis, J. R. (1969). A shunt operation for obesity. *Dis. Colon. Rectum*, **12**, 115

48 Wills, C. E. (1971). Obstetrical delivery after jejuno-ileostomy for obesity. *J. Med. Ass. Georgia*, **60**, 39

49 Payne, J. H., DeWind, L. T., Schwab, C. E. and Kern, W. H. (1973). Surgical treatment of morbid obesity. Sixteen years of experience. *Arch. Surg.*, **106**, 432

50 Olow, B., Akesson, B. A., Dencker, H., Green, A. and Norryd, C. (1976). Pregnancy after jejuno-ileostomy because of obesity. *Acta. Chir. Scand.*, **142**, 82

51 Fielding, J. W. L. and Baddeley, R. M. (1978). The effect of small bowel bypass on diabetes mellitus. *Br. J. Surg.*, **65**, 30

52 Scott, H. W., Dean, R., Younger, R. K. and Butte, W. H. (1974). Changes in hyperlipidaemia and hyperlipoproteinaemia in morbidly obese patients treated by jejuno-ileal bypass. *Surg. Gynecol. Obstet.*, **138**, 353

53 Shibata, H. R., Mackenzie, J. R. and Long, R. (1967). Metabolic effects of controlled jejunocolic bypass. *Arch. Surg.*, **95**, 413

54 Benfield, J. R., Greenway, F. L., Bray, G. A., Barry, R. E., Lechago, J., Mena, I. and Schedewie, H. (1976). Experience with jejuno-ileal bypass for obesity. *Surg. Gynecol. Obstet.*, **143**, 401

55 Bendezu, F., Wieland, R. G., Green, S. G., Hallberg, M. C. and Masters, R. W. (1976). Certain metabolic consequences of jejuno-ileal bypass. *Am. J. Clin. Nutr.*, **29**, 366

56 Moore, R. B., Frantz, I. D. and Buchwald, H. (1969). Changes in cholesterol pool size turnover rate, and faecal bile acid and sterol excretion after partial ileal bypass in hypercholesterolaemic patients. *Surgery*, **65**, 98

57 Wise, L. and Stein, T. (1975). Biliary and urinary calculi – pathogenesis following small bowel bypass for obesity. *Arch. Surg.*, **110**, 1043

58 Buchwald, H. Varco, R. L., Moore, R. B. and Schwartz, M. Z. (1975). Intestinal bypass procedures, partial ileal bypass for hyperlipidaemia and jejuno-ileal bypass for obesity. In M. M. Ravitch (ed.). *Current Problems in Surgery*. (Chicago: Year Book Medical Publishers)

59 Johnson, C. D. and Bynum, T. E. (1976). Hypocalcaemia as a complication of jejuno-ileal bypass for morbid obesity. *Sth. Med. J.*, **69**, 616

60 Dano, P. and Christiansen, C. (1974). Calcium absorption and bone mineral contents following intestinal shunt operation in obesity. *Scand. J. Gastroenterol*, **9**, 775

61 Scott, H. W., Dean, R. H., Shull, H. J., Abram, H. S., Younger, R. K. and Brill, A. B. (1973). New considerations in use of jejuno-ileal bypass in patients with morbid obesity. *Ann. Surg.*, **177**, 723

62 Moxley, R. T., Pozefsky, T. and Lockwood, D. H. (1974). Protein nutrition and liver disease after jejuno-ileal bypass for morbid obesity. *N. Engl. J. Med.*, **290**, 921

63 Kern, W. H., Heger, A. H., Payne, J. H. and DeWind, L. T. (1973). Fatty metamorphosis of the liver in morbid obesity. *Arch. Pathol.*, **96**, 342

64 Dano, P., Nielson, O. V., Petri, M. and Jorgensen, B. (1975). Liver morphology and liver function before and after intestinal shunt operation for obesity. *Scand. J. Gastroenterol.*, **10**, 409

65 Salmon, P. A. and Reedyk, L. (1975). Fatty metamorphosis in patients with jejuno-ileal bypass. *Surg. Gynecol. Obstet.*, **141**, 75

66 Marubbio, A. T., Buchwald, H., Schwartz, M. Z. and Varco, R. L. (1976). Hepatic lesions of central pericellular fibrosis in morbid obesity and after jejuno-ileal bypass. *Am. J. Clin. Path.*, **66**, 684

67 Buchwald, H., Lober, P. H. and Varco, R. L. (1974). Liver biopsy findings in seventy-seven consecutive patients undergoing jejuno-ileal bypass for morbid obesity. *Am. J. Surg.*, **127**, 48

68 Holzbach, R. T. (1977). Hepatic effects of jejuno-ileal bypass for morbid obesity. *Am. J. Clin. Nutr.*, **30**, 43

69 Soyer, M. T., Ceballos, R. and Aldrete, J. S. (1976). Reversibility of severe hepatic damage caused by jejuno-ileal bypass after re-establishment of normal intestinal continuity. *Surgery*, **79**, 601

70 Mangla, J. C., Hoy, W., Kim, Y. and Chopek, M. (1974). Cirrhosis and death after jejuno-ileal shunt for obesity. *Am. J. Dig. Dis.*, **19**, 759

71 McGill, D. B., Humphreys, S. R., Baggenstoss, A. U. and Dickson, E. R. (1972). Cirrhosis and death after jejuno-ileal shunt. *Gastroenterology*, **63**, 872

72 Heimburger, S. L., Steiger, E., Gerfo, P. L., Bichl, A. G. and Williams, M. J. (1975). Reversal of severe fatty hepatic infiltration after intestinal bypass for morbid obesity by calorie free amino-acid infusion. *Am. J. Surg.*, **129**, 229

73 Ames, F. C., Copeland, E. M., Leeb, D. C. *et al.* (1976). Liver dysfunction following small bowel bypass for obesity: non-operative treatment of fatty metamorphosis with parenteral hyperalimentation. *J. Am. Med. Ass.*, **235**, 1249

74 Lockwood, D. H., Amatruda, J. M., Moxley, R. T., Pozefsky, T. and Boitnott, J. K. (1977). Effect of oral amino acid supplementation on liver disease after jejuno-ileal bypass for morbid obesity. *Am. J. Clin. Nutr.*, **30**, 58

75 White, J. J., Moxley, R. T., Pozefsky, T. and Lockwood, D. H. (1974). Transient kwashiorkor: a cause of fatty liver following small bowel bypass. *Surgery*, **75**, 829

76 Hoyumpa, A. M., Greene, H. L., Dunn, G. D. (1975). Fatty liver: biochemical and clinical consideration. *Am. J. Dig. Dis.*, **20**, 1142

77 Sherr, H. P., Nair, P. P., White, J. J., Banwell, J. G. and Lockwood, D. H. (1974). Bile acid metabolism and hepatic disease following small bowel bypass for obesity. *Am. J. Clin. Nutr.*, **27**, 1369

78 Drenick, E. J., Simmons, F. and Murphy, J. F. (1970). Effect on hepatic morphology of treatment of obesity by fasting reducing diets and small bowel bypass. *N. Engl. J. Med.*, **282**, 829

79 Peters, R. L., Gay, T. and Reynolds, T. B. (1975). Post jejuno-ileal bypass hepatic disease. Its similarity to alcholic hepatic disease. *Am. J. Clin. Path.*, **63**, 318

80 Mezey, E., Imbenbo, A. L., Potter, J. J., Rent, K. C., Lombardo, R. and Holt, P. R. (1975). Endogenous ethanol production and hepatic disease following jejuno-ileal bypass for morbid obesity. *Am. J. Clin. Nutr.*, **28,** 1277

81 Passaro, E., Drenick, E. and Wilson, S. E. (1976). Bypass enteritis: a new complication of jejuno-ileal bypass for obesity. *Am. J. Surg.*, **131,** 169

82 Menguy, R. (1976). Pneumatosis intestinalis after jejuno-ileal bypass. *J. Am. Med. Ass.*, **236,** 1721

83 Martyak, S. N. and Curtis, L. E. (1976). Pneumatosis intestinalis: a complication of jejunal-ileal bypass. *J. Am. Med. Ass.*, **235,** 1038

84 Saunders, G. B. (1977). Bypass enteritis or obstructive volvulus. *Arch. Surg.*, **112,** 668

85 Shagrin, J. W., Frane, B. and Duncan, H. (1971). Polyarthritis in obese patients with intestinal bypass. *Ann. Intern. Med.*, **75,** 377

86 Hess, R. J. (1974). Polyarthritis after small bowel bypass. *J. Oklahoma State Med. Ass.*, **67,** 283

87 Mir-Majdlessi, S. H., Mackenzie, A. H. and Winkelman, E. I. (1974). Articular complications in obese patients after jejunocolic bypass. *Cleveland Clin. Quart.*, **41,** 119

88 Wands, J. R., Lamont, J. T., Mann, E. and Isselbacher, K. H. (1976). Arthritis associated with intestinal bypass procedure for morbid obesity. *N. Engl. J. Med.*, **294,** 121

89 Earnest, D. L. (1977). Perspectives on incidence, aetiology and treatment of enteric hyperoxaluria. *Am. J. Clin. Nutr.*, **30,** 72

90 Cryer, P. E., Garber, A. J., Hoffsten, P., Lucas, B. and Wise, L. (1975). Renal failure after small intestinal bypass for obesity. *Arch. Intern. Med.*, **135,** 1610

91 Bennison, L. J. and Grundy, S. M. (1975). Effects of obesity and calorie intake on biliary lipid metabolism in man. *J. Clin. Invest.*, **56,** 996

92 Freeman, J. B., Mayer, P. D., Printent, K. J., Mason, E. E. and Denbestre, L. (1975). Analysis of gall bladder bile in morbid obesity. *Am. J. Surg.*, **129,** 163

93 Barry, R. E., Barisch, J., Bray, G. A., Sperling, M. A., Mopin, R. J. and Benfield, J. (1977). Intestinal adaptation after jejuno-ileal bypass in man. *Am. J. Clin. Nutr.*, **30,** 32

94 Morin, R. J., and Barry, R. E. (1976). Lipid composition of bile before and after jejuno-ileal bypass surgery. *Clin. Chim. Acta.*, **69,** 479

95 Dano, P., Lenz, K. and Justesen, T. (1974). Bile acid metabolism and intestinal bacterial flora after three types of intestinal shunt operation for obesity. *Scand. J. Gastroenterol.*, **9,** 767

96 Neshat, A. A. and Flye, M. W. (1975). Early formation of gallstones following jejuno-ileal bypass for treatment of morbid obesity. *Am. Surg.*, **41,** 486

97 Barry, R. E., Benfield, J. R., Nicell, P. and Bray, G. A. (1975). Colonic pseudo obstruction: a new complication of jejuno-ileal bypass. *Gut*, **16,** 903

98 Juhl, E., Brunsgaad, A., Hippe, Korner, B., Quaade, F., Baden, H. (1974). Vitamin B_{12} depletion in obese patients treated with jejuno-ileal anastomosis. *Scand. J. Gastroenterol.*, **9,** 543

99 Dano, P. and Lenz, K. (1974). Change in bile acid metabolism and absorption of Vitamin B_{12} after intestinal shunt operation in obesity. *Scand. J. Gastroenterol.*, **9,** 159

100 Mason, E. E, and Ito, G. (1969). Gastric bypass in obesity. *Surg. Clin. N. Amer.*, **47,** 1345

101 Mason, E. E. and Ito, C. (1969). Gastric bypass, *Ann. Surg.*, **170,** 329

102 Printen, K. J. and Mason, E. E. (1973). Gastric surgery for relief of morbid obesity. *Arch. Surg.*, **106,** 428

103 Printen, K. J. and Mason, E. E. (1977). Gastric bypass for morbid obesity in patients more than 50 years of age. *Surg. Gynecol. Obstet.*, **144,** 192

104 Soper, R. T., Mason, E. E., Printen, K. J. and Zellmeger, H. (1975). Gastric bypass for morbid obesity in children and adolescents. *J. Paediatr. Surg.*, **10,** 51

105 Hornberger, H. R. (1976). Gastric bypass. *Am. J. Surg.*, **131,** 415

106 Griffen, W. O., Young, V. L. and Stevenson, C. C. (1977). A prospective comparison of gastric and jejuno-ileal bypass procedures for morbid obesity. *Ann. Surg.*, **186,** 500

107 Hitchcock, C. T., Jewell, W. R., Hardin, C. A., and Hermreck, A. S. (1977). Management of the morbidly obese patient after small bowel bypass failure. *Surgery*, **82,** 356

108 Sorrell, V. F. and Burcher, S. K. (1976). Gastric bypass for morbid obesity. *N.Z. Med. J.*, **84,** 96

109 Hermreck, A. S., Jewell, W. R. and Hardin, C. R. (1976). Gastric bypass for morbid obesity. *Surg. Gynecol. Obstet.*, **80,** 498

110 Alden, J. F. (1977). Gastric and jejuno-ileal bypass. *Arch. Surg.*, **112,** 799

111 Mason, E. E., Printen, K. J., Hartford, C. E. and Boyd, W. C. (1975). Optimising results of gastric bypass. *Ann. Surg.*, **182,** 405

112 Mason, E. E., Munns, J. R., Kealey, G. P., Wangler, R., Clarke, W. R., Cheng, H. F. and Printen, K. J. (1976). Effect of gastric bypass on gastric secretion. *Am. J. Surg.*, **131,** 162

113 Wood, G. D. (1977). The early results of treatment of the obese by a diet regime enforced by maxillo mandibular fixation. *J. Oral. Surg.*, **35,** 461

114 Rodgers, S., Goss, A., Goldney, R., Thomas, D., Burnett, R., Phillips, P., Kimber, C. and Harding, P. (1977). Jaw wiring in treatment of obesity. *Lancet*, **ii,** 1221

115 Garrow, J. S. (1973). Diet and obesity. *Proc. Roy. Soc. Med.*, **66,** 642

8

Behaviour therapy and self-help programmes for obesity

A. J. Stunkard and K. D. Brownell

INTRODUCTION

The two most promising new approaches to management of mild to moderate obesity are behaviour therapy and non-professional weight reduction groups. Combining these two modalities would seem a particularly felicitous strategy; one study has now shown that introducing behavioural methods into a non-professional group can significantly improve its performance[1]. This chapter deals with these two new approaches.

The obese have not been at a loss to find treatments that promise weight loss as well as happiness, improved relations with the opposite sex, and increased self-confidence. A glance into almost any popular magazine turns up advertisements promoting cures for obesity; most are untested at best, dangerous at worst.

Why is there such a booming market for weight reduction methods? The answer seems clear: millions are plagued by excess weight. Many attempt to reduce by methods that are largely ineffective. Confronted by failure, they move on to another approach and then another, creating a lucrative business for those who promise what cannot be delivered. The fact that so many overweight people are attracted to such questionable measures is testimony to how desperately they want to lose weight and how difficult it is for them to do so. Millions more have given up even trying.

Little more than 15 years ago the results of treatment programmes for obesity were particularly discouraging: 'Most obese persons will not enter treatment for obesity. Of those who enter treatment, most will not lose weight, and of those who do lose weight, most will regain it'[2]. These were harsh words, indeed. What was their basis?

The proportion of obese people who enter treatment is still uncertain, but it clearly varies with social status: young upper-middle-class women

199

probably diet frequently, lower-class persons of both sexes probably diet rarely.

There is a great deal of information on attrition rates in routine medical treatment for obesity and these rates are high; one survey has placed them at 20–80%[3]. A particularly instructive example is illustrated in Figure 1.

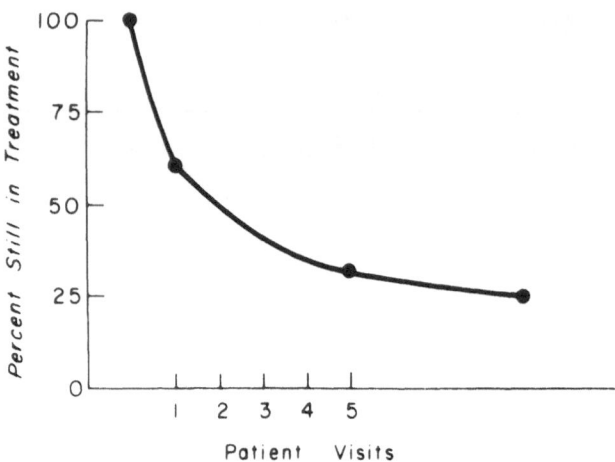

Figure 1 Attrition rate of 151 persons during outpatient treatment for obesity. Adapted from Shipman[4]

This figure was constructed from data in a report designed, ironically, to support the view that weight reduction in routine medical treatment is relatively effective and is achieved without any great distress[4]. Such favourable results may well have been achieved by the 20% who persevered.

Of the patients who do remain in treatment, most lose little weight. The aforementioned survey revealed that fewer than 25% of those in outpatient therapy lost as much as 20 lb (9·1 kg) and only 5% lost as much as 40 lb (18·2 kg)[3]. Another survey, which involved more elaborate analyses, indicated similarly discouraging results[5–6].

Data on follow-up are sparse, but the few available are revealing. In one report of routine medical management of obesity, only 12 out of 100 patients lost as much as 20 lb (9·1 kg); a year later only two of these 12 had maintained their weight[3].

Nor do these findings end our tale of woe; it is a sad fact that many obese persons suffer painful emotional reactions to routine attempts at medical methods of weight reduction. A recent review has confirmed that emotional symptoms occur in about 50% of persons treated for obesity, whether by outpatient dieting or inpatient fasting[7]. In 1967, a short report by Richard Stuart on 'Behavioral Control of Overeating', was in dramatic contrast to this unrelieved picture of failure[8]. Stuart described the best results in the outpatient treatment of obesity reported up to that time. His paper was a landmark in our understanding of this disorder.

Stuart's results, summarized in Figures 2 and 3, show the weight losses, over a 1-year period, of the eight patients who remained in treatment out of

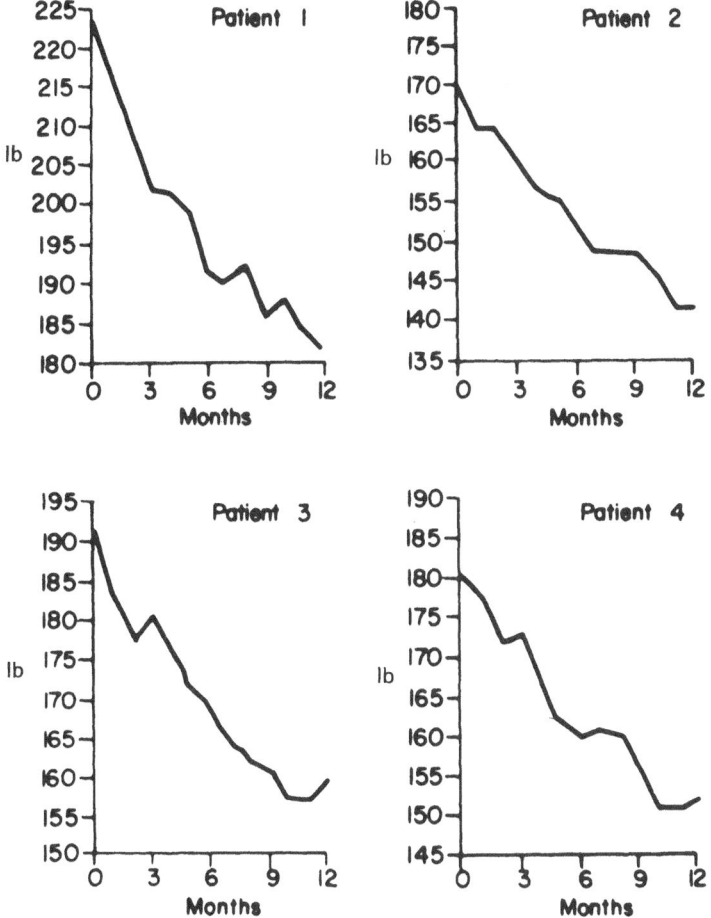

Figure 2 Weight losses of four women receiving behavioural treatment for obesity. From Stuart[8]

an original ten. Three, or 30%, lost more than 40 lb (18·2 kg) and 60% lost more than 30 lb (13·6 kg). Certain features of the report deserve attention. First, the expenditure of time was not exorbitant. In fact, time spent in treatment was no greater than that in a number of studies showing far poorer results. At the beginning of the treatment period, patients were seen in 30 min sessions held three times a week, for a total of 12 to 15 sessions.

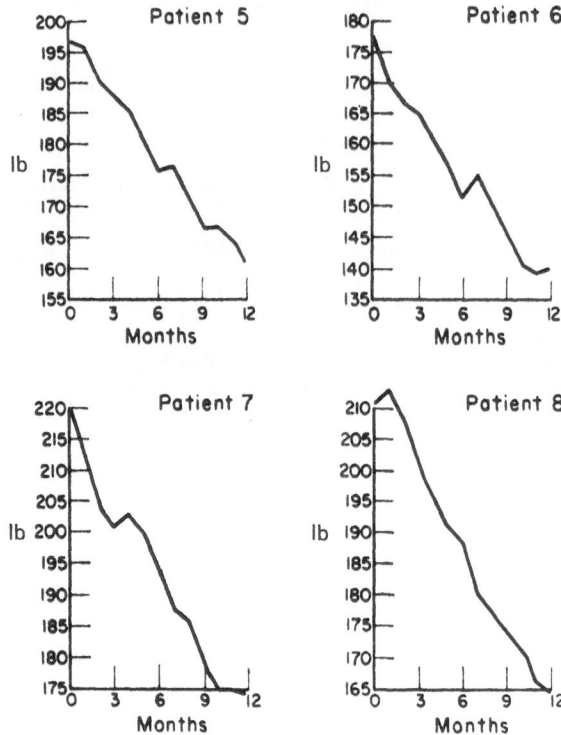

Figure 3 Weight losses of four women receiving behavioural treatment for obesity. From Stuart[8]

Thereafter, treatment sessions were scheduled as needed, usually at 2-week intervals, for the next 3 months. Subsequently, patients had weekly sessions and, finally, 'maintenance' sessions as needed. The total number of visits during the year varied from 16 to 41.

There was no evidence of the 'symptom substitution' that psychodynamically oriented theorists have warned against, and seven of the eight patients reported that they had developed an increased range of social activities. Three of the six married patients reported more satisfying relationships with their spouses. Furthermore, three of the eight who were also heavy smokers applied the same kind of behavioural approach and either substantially reduced or stopped smoking. Clearly a new dimension had been added to the outpatient treatment of obesity.

It was not long before this approach attracted the attention of research workers and in the decade since the publication of Stuart's original paper there has been an explosion of research on behavioural control of obesity. Over 100 papers have appeared, marked by increasingly sophisticated methodology. No fewer than six long review articles and several books have described this development in recent years[9-16].

The programme Stuart used in this and in a later, comparably effective study[17] was based on an earlier largely theoretical report by Ferster *et al.*[18]. The work of Stuart and Ferster has influenced behavioural treatment programmes. It is appropriate at this time to consider the programme in detail along with refinements recently added. More detailed accounts are provided in a book by the Mahoneys[19] and a manual by Ferguson[20].

A DESCRIPTION OF THE BEHAVIOURAL PROGRAMME

The behavioural programme can be divided into four sections; (1) measurement and description of eating behaviours; (2) modification of the antecedents of eating behaviour; (3) modification of the act of eating itself; and (4) modification of the consequences of eating. Within each category, there are at least a dozen behaviours that will be prescribed in a typical programme. In this section we will describe the rationale and a few sample behaviours.

Measurement of eating behaviour: self-monitoring

Self-monitoring is usually the first behaviour to be prescribed. It involves having the patient make a careful record of body weight, caloric intake, physical activity, and any factors that may influence eating (e.g., emotional states and social interactions). Most importantly, as the programme progresses, patients are asked to monitor the behaviours they are asked to change. In most programmes subjects are given convenient recording forms, and the information from these forms can provide means by which changes in behaviour can be reinforced by the therapist, or the patient him/herself.

Initially self-monitoring was used as an information-gathering procedure to evaluate an individual's eating patterns and suggest where changes were to be made. However, self-monitoring was sometimes reactive, altering the very behaviour it was to measure. This finding prompted some behaviour therapists to view self-monitoring as a valid therapeutic procedure[21]. Subsequent studies have shown that self-monitoring cannot stand alone as a treatment for the obese[22-24], but is important to include in the total package[19].

Self-monitoring is useful both for the therapist and the patient because it yields a picture of an individual's eating patterns. Such a picture allows the therapist to tailor the treatment techniques to the patient's needs. In addition, recording a behaviour can highlight patterns that had gone unnoticed. For example, many obese people eat 'automatically' and are unaware of the amount they consume. Most are genuinely surprised when looking at self-recording charts for the first days of a behavioural programme. Self-monitoring also provides a measure against which patients can evaluate their performance.

Some research has been conducted to determine methods for increasing the accuracy and reactivity of self-monitoring. It is helpful to provide a convenient recording form and to be certain that completing it is reinforced by the health professional. Patients are encouraged to record the behaviour immediately after it occurs, because accuracy and reactivity decline with time. As previously mentioned, patients are instructed to record the feelings and events that surround eating, and to record component behaviours (prescribed eating behaviours) as well as movement toward the target goal (weight change).

Altering the antecedents: stimulus control

One focus of a behavioural analysis is the constellation of variables that precede eating. If particular events always occur before eating, it is possible that modifying these events can aid in gaining control over the act of eating. Stimulus control, or cue elimination, behaviours are prescribed for this purpose. Patients are encouraged to keep all food in the house out of sight, to keep high-calorie foods out of the house, and to limit the accessibility of food that must be kept in the house. Candy and nut dishes are to be eliminated, and when visitors arrive, low-calorie foods are to be served. Foods that require preparation (raw vegetables, soups, etc.) are to replace those that are prepared (e.g., potato chips). Patients are to carry little spare change so that impulse-buying, as from candy machines, can be reduced.

Programmes have also concentrated on behaviour patterns that may become cues to signal eating. Many overweight people report eating when watching television. When this occurs frequently enough, the television may become a signal to eat, regardless of whether the person is hungry. The same phenomenon can occur at specific times of the day, in specific locations, and while engaging in specific activities. Therefore, patients are instructed to minimize the number of times, places, and events associated with eating. They are asked to do nothing else while eating, to eat in a specific place, and to eat only at scheduled times. In order to develop new stimuli associated with appropriate eating behaviours, patients are encouraged to have a specific eating place in their homes and even to use a distinctive table setting as a cue.

Controlling the act of eating

Behavioural programmes attempt to bring the act of eating under the patient's control. This involves allowing the rate of eating and increasing awareness of the components of the eating process. Patients are to put their forks down between each bite and to pause in mid-meal. Originally designed to interrupt the automatic chain of eating behaviours (lifting the fork, putting food into the mouth, etc.), this also serves to postpone a portion of the meal until such time as the absorption of food has begun to produce physiological signals of satiety. There is some controversy about whether the obese eat faster than the non-obese, but slowing the rate of eating is probably a useful strategy even if they do not.

Patients are also asked to try to make eating an enjoyable experience by concentrating on each bite and to make meals a time for relaxation and comfort. The hope is that a smaller amount of food will provide adequate enjoyment if each bite is appreciated to its fullest. Interestingly, many patients report truly enjoying food for the first time. They become aware that at times in the past they have consumed extraordinary amounts of food (e.g., an entire pie) without tasting it. The fact that people enjoy their food more may partially explain why there are fewer dropouts from behaviour therapy than from traditional therapies.

Modifying the consequences of eating

One of the principles of learning theory is that behaviour must be reinforced if it is to be maintained. Over-eating presents a particular problem in this respect. The rewards of this inappropriate behaviour are immediate and powerful, whereas punishment (increased risk of cardiovascular disease, ridicule, etc.) is remote. Conversely, the rewards for adhering to a dietary regimen are remote and the sacrifice immediate. This reinforcement/ punishment inbalance must be modified for weight loss to occur. Behavioural programmes have used several procedures to accomplish this. First, group leaders use social pressures to reinforce behaviour changes and weight changes. In some programmes, family members are instructed to do the same[25-27]. It is important to note that separate systems can be established to reward weight change and to reward behaviour change. Of the two, behaviour change appears to be the more important. This is consistent with the notion that weight changes are not likely to be maintained if new eating behaviours are not developed.

For some patients, a system of more tangible and self-administered rewards is helpful. In such a system, the patient makes a list of the relevant behaviours to be followed. Points or tokens are awarded for adherence to the programme, and then 'cashed in' for back-up reinforcers: going to the films, buying a new dress, reading a magazine, etc. For some, earning the points serves as an indication of progress and the back-up reinforcements are not necessary.

Programmes have experimented with having the rewards controlled by the therapist (contingency contracting) or by the patient. In a contingency contracting system, the patient contracts with the therapist that certain behaviours will be exchanged for rewards or avoidance of punishments. The therapist serves as a resource and consults with the patient in the development of the contingency system. One study compared the effectiveness of a self-controlled system with that of an externally controlled system[28]. Although the findings are not definitive, it appears that self-controlled rewards may be more effective. Whatever the system, it is important that rewards and/or points be dispensed as soon as possible after the behaviour occurs.

Other components of the behavioural programme

Several components recently have been added to the basics of the Stuart programme. An important one is cognitive restructuring. This addition was the result of behaviour therapists' interest in the thoughts and cognitions that influence behaviour[29, 30], and their realization that overweight people often have maladaptive thoughts that impede their progress through a dieting programme. Mahoney and Mahoney[19, 26] have put forth a programme of cognitive restructuring for the obese, which they call 'cleaning up the cognitive ecology'. They have highlighted five types of self-defeating cognitions and have outlined counter-statements to be used by the dieter. Simple repetition of the counter-statements may be useful even if the patient does not completely believe them at first. After all, their own irrational and self-destructive statements have become 'fact' to the patient, even though they might have seemed ridiculous at the outset.

Here are examples of the five types of statements the present authors have heard from the obese, along with counter-arguments:

(1) *Weight:* 'It's taking forever to lose weight. I guess this means I will be fat forever.' A counter-argument is, 'I am losing slowly but surely, and this time I will learn how to keep it off.'

(2) *Capabilities:* 'I've never been able to lose much weight before. Why should it work this time?' A counter-argument is, 'Maybe this will be the first time; and don't forget, this time I have some powerful procedures going for me.'

(3) *Excuses:* 'Everyone in my family has had a weight problem. It must be my genes.' A counter-argument is, 'That may make it harder, but not impossible. If I stick with the programme, I will succeed.'

(4) *Goals:* 'I will never eat chocolate cake again, and that will help me lose weight fast.' A counter-argument is, 'These are unrealistic expectations and when I don't live up to them I will only get discouraged. I should pay more attention to the eating behaviours I have been learning.'

(5) *Food thoughts:* 'I can just taste how good that ice cream will be.' A useful response would be, 'STOP THAT! I should think of something to do that will take me away from thoughts of eating.'

It may also be important to discuss the likelihood of relapses, and to be prepared to deal with them when they occur. Many obese people feel they are either 'on' a diet or 'off' a diet. Therefore, if they stray from their self-imposed dieting boundaries, any number of self-defeating cognitions can ensue, i.e., 'This proves that I am a fat slob and that I have no willpower'. Preparing patients for these thoughts can improve performance during difficult times.

Exercise is another component of some behavioural programmes, and one which the authors feel is important. The benefits of regular exercise on cardiovascular fitness and body weight have been clearly documented[31]. Therefore, regular and rigorous exercise routines are indicated for obese people, if their physical condition permits. Unfortunately, few can be counted on to devote themselves to such a routine and overweight people (as well as many slim people) report that such a regimen of swimming, cycling, etc. is tedious, time-consuming, painful, and most importantly, difficult to maintain. Therefore, we have been concentrating on routine exercise or the amount of activity that can be programmed into a person's daily routine. A recent study[32] discovered that obese people are five times less likely than people of normal weight to choose the stairs rather than escalators in public places. The behavioural programmes attempt to overcome this sedentary behaviour by instructing patients to make use of opportunities for small increases in physical activity: using the stairs more often, parking some distance from their destination, getting off the bus one stop early, etc. These behaviours are monitored and reinforced, and become an integral part of the programme.

BEHAVIOUR THERAPY AND OBESITY: NATURAL PARTNERS

Within the past two decades, behaviour therapy has been the object of a dramatic increase in interest. Many investigators have focused on outcome research, and treatment of obesity has become a popular proving ground for the evaluation of behavioural self-control procedures. As Wilson has pointed out, obesity, unlike most other clinical problems, offers 'a definitive yet convenient and objective measure of outcome efficacy – weight reduction'[10]. Investigators have also been influenced by the fact that the obese provide readily available subject populations. These factors have resulted in much research into obesity, and have taught us a great deal in the past several years. In this section we will outline the development of behaviour therapy for obesity and will highlight the well-designed studies that have contributed to the birth of a new behavioural programme.

Scrutiny of behavioural programmes: methodological advances
In the mid-1960s and early 1970s behavioural researchers were making

their mark by subjecting psychotherapeutic procedures to rigorous experimental evaluation. Paul's study on systematic desensitization was used as a model for many treatment outcome studies of a number of disorders[33]. The treatment of obesity has been central in this movement.

The first step was to move beyond Stuart's first, uncontrolled study. Stuart's findings had left unanswered the question of whether the same subjects would have lost weight if untreated, or if treated with different procedures. Harris[34] addressed the first question by randomly assigning 24 overweight subjects to two behavioural treatment groups, or to a control group that received no treatment. Subjects first were treated in groups twice weekly, then less frequently for a 10-week treatment period, and were weighed at the end of a 16-week follow-up period. Subjects given behavioural treatment lost significantly more weight than did control subjects, and perhaps most important, continued to lose weight after the treatment sessions had ended. Also, Harris's study highlighted the viability of treating overweight people in groups. Mean weight loss for the behavioural groups in this study was 10·5 lb (4·8 kg), far below what Stuart had found. This may have resulted from the fact that Harris's subjects were far less obese than those of Stuart, and she treated them for a far shorter period of time. Her use of a group *versus* Stuart's individual treatment did not seem to be responsible, since a well-controlled study has shown group treatment to be *more* effective than individual treatment[35].

At this point it was evident that behavioural treatment was better than no treatment; but the method had not been compared to other treatments. In 1970, Wollersheim published a study that compared behaviour therapy to another therapy, and also to a placebo control[36]. Subjects were assigned to four regimes:

1. Behaviour therapy (focal therapy);
2. Non-specific therapy to control for therapist attention, with presentation of a treatment rationale. This group focused on the 'underlying reasons' and 'unconscious motives' underlying their personality;
3. Social pressure therapy, based on the commercial self-help group TOPS (Take Off Pounds Sensibly) and involving group praise and encouragement; and
4. A no-treatment control group.

Four therapists treated one group of five subjects in each regime for a total of ten sessions over a 3-month treatment period. Subjects were weighed at the end of a 2 month follow-up period. At post-treatment and at 2-month follow-up, those in the behavioural condition had lost significantly more weight than had those in the no-treatment regime, and also than those in the other regimes (see Figure 4). This suggested that behavioural procedures were effective over and above the effects to be expected when

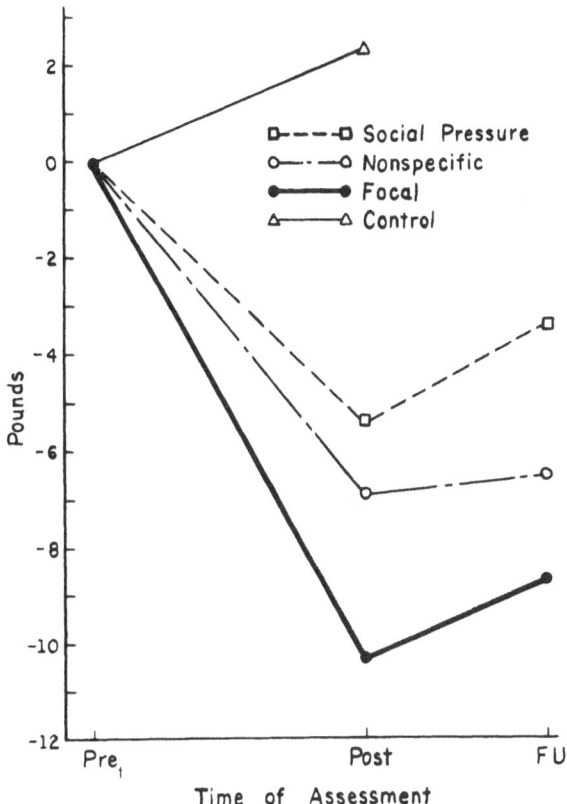

Figure 4 Mean weight losses in pounds of the focal (behavioural) group, the two alternative treatment control groups, and the no-treatment control group. From Wollersheim[36]

individuals benefit from the social factors inherent in receiving any treatment.

Wollersheim's study represented a significant methodological advance in the study of obesity in particular and of behaviour change in general; and it brought such research face to face for the first time with a traditional problem – experimenter bias. For although Wollersheim's placebo treatments controlled for the patients' expectations of treatment, they could not control for the therapists', and this is hardly a trivial matter. In large measure, therapeutic effectiveness must surely depend on the therapist's expectations. The double-blind experiment in psychopharmacology has shown how powerful this influence can be when medication is concerned. It is surely more powerful in the more emotional psychotherapies. Therapists' expectations of the efficacy of behavioural treatment must have been

The Treatment of Obesity

at a peak in the behaviourally oriented department at the University of Illinois, where Wollersheim conducted her research.

It is unlikely that the behavioural researcher will ever attain the elegance and economy of the psychopharmacologist's double-blind methodology. Controlling experimenter bias will require methods tailored to the special needs and opportunities of this kind of research. One such method, deceptively simple, was introduced by Penick et al. [37].

The essence of this ingenious method was to give up at the start the notion that therapists could be unbiased in the use of therapies they favoured or disfavoured. Instead, therapists were selected on the basis of their commitment to a particular approach. Penick biased the outcome against the behavioural approach by selecting therapists of vastly different experience for the two regimes. For the behavioural treatment, the therapists were beginners; for the control group they were experts.

Subjects were treated in groups for sessions of 2 hours over a 3-month period. The results revealed that patients treated behaviourally lost more weight than did those treated with the entire traditional therapeutic

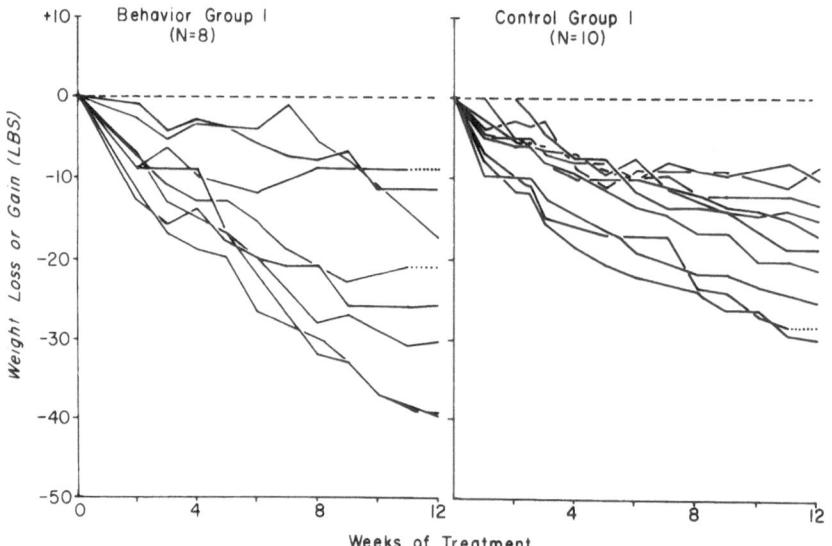

Figure 5 Individual weight changes in pounds of severely obese persons receiving behaviour therapy or control therapy – subjects from one cohort. From Penick et al. [37]

armamentarium. Finally, the Penick study[37] showed that behaviour modification, even when delivered by a team with little experience, was more effective against obesity than was the best alternative programme that a research team with long experience in treatment of the disorder could devise (see Figures 5 and 6).

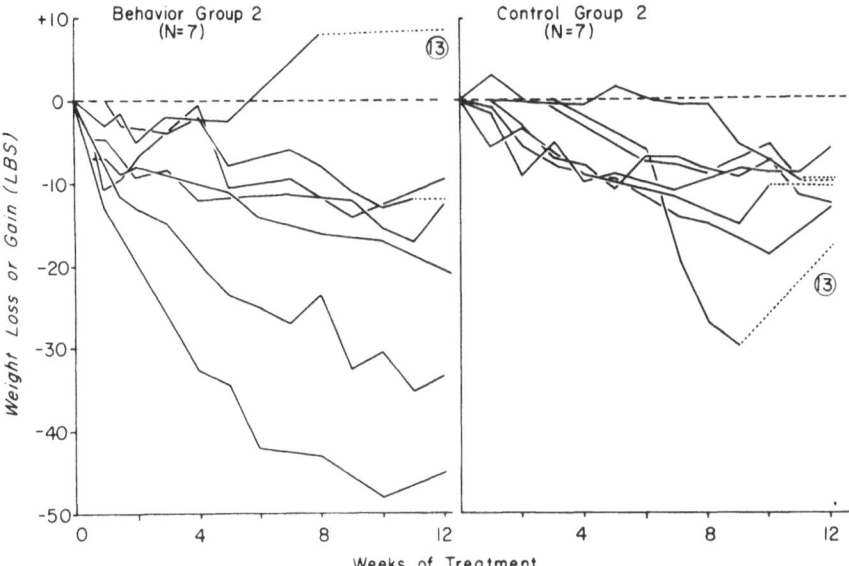

Figure 6 Individual weight changes in pounds of severely obese persons in Penick *et al.'s* second cohort. From Penick *et al.*[37]

This result flies in the face of one of psychotherapy's beliefs that the personal characteristics and experience of the psychotherapist are more important than is the nature of the psychotherapy. The Penick study suggested instead that the content of the behavioural programme outweighed these characteristics of the therapists, and provided a new type of evidence for the efficacy of a behavioural approach. It also suggested a radical new approach to obesity: therapy without a therapist.

Therapy without a therapist
If the content of the behavioural programme is more important than the characteristics of the therapist, is it possible that this content actually could substitute for the personal influence of the therapist? In 1974, Richard Hagen apparently answered the question in the affirmative[38]. He compared an exact replication of Wollershiem's behavioural programme as carried out by a therapist with what he called 'bibliotherapy,' which consisted of a manual of ten lessons mailed at weekly intervals to the participating subjects. The manual, constructed from that used by the therapists in Wollersheim's first treatment condition, took the form of a programmed text, with homework assignments that the subjects mailed back each week to the investigator, who corrected them and returned them to the subjects. A third treatment group, manual plus therapist contact, also offered lessons

on a 10-week basis, but the exchange of lessons and of homework took place at the treatment sessions, not by mail.

Hagen's 90 subjects were mildly (25%) overweight university students, randomly assigned to one of the three treatment regimes or to a no-treatment control group. Ten treatment sessions were held over a 3-month period.

The 'contact only' and bibliotherapy groups produced identical weight losses – an average of 12 lb (5·5 kg), which was not significantly different from the average loss of 15 lb (6·8 kg) for the contact plus bibliotherapy regime. Hagen exuberantly concluded, 'the present investigation demonstrates that it is possible to treat obesity effectively using a written manual, and that this treatment is apparently as effective as any yet evaluated in a controlled study.... In terms of practical significance, the findings ... point to the possibility of offering an effective treatment for obesity without the involvement of costly and scarce professional time.' Ferstl *et al.* at the Max Planck Institute in Munich[39] found remarkably similar results under quite different conditions. They compared a 'broad spectrum behavioural programme' with strong emphasis on stimulus control, administered by therapists, with the identical programme administered by 'letter therapy'. Forty persons, mainly women, averaging 30% overweight, were randomly assigned to either programme. These programmes consisted of a 2-week baseline period followed by 10 weeks of active treatment, a 5-week interval without treatment, and a final 2-week treatment period. Therapy was unusually intrusive, occurring twice a week and, in the contact regime, was carried out by two therapists who treated groups of no more than five subjects each. Weight loss in the contact regime averaged 17 lb (7·7 kg), and that in the 'letter therapy' condition, 16 lb (7·3 kg), a difference that was far from statistically significant.

A third study, which found no difference between subjects treated by conventional face-to-face behaviour therapy and those who received a programmed text and little professional contact, was carried out by Hanson, Borden, Hall and Hall[40]. Face-to-face subjects lost an average of 7·9% of initial body weight over the 10 weeks of treatment, compared to a weight loss of 5·4% of initial body weight by the bibliotherapy subjects. As is usual in such studies, even these modest weight losses were not maintained.

In contrast to the three foregoing studies, Brownell *et al.*[41] *did* find a difference between face-to-face treatment and bibliotherapy, the former subjects losing 10·3 lb (4·7 kg), and the latter 4·3 lb (2·0 kg). Again weight losses were not maintained; at 6-month follow-up, differences between the treatments had disappeared.

These studies have been as important for the theoretical and methodological issues they have raised as for their practical results. The study of psychological treatment could be greatly advanced if it were possible to treat people without professional contact, for the greatest source of uncontrolled variance – the influence of the therapist – would be eliminated; and it would become possible to study various forms of treatment in large numbers of people at very low cost. Furthermore, it might make it possible to determine more precisely the effect of the therapist's personal influence. Personal contact of varying intensity and character could be introduced into bibliotherapy and the effects observed. Just this kind of study was carried out with instructive results by Fernan[42].

Inspired by a supervisor who had participated in Hagen's pioneering bibliography study, Fernan compared the effectiveness of bibliotherapy when conducted in the context of two levels of therapist involvement. One level had minimal involvement (such as was described in Hagen's report) confined to comments on the written records that the patients mailed to him and which he returned. The second, higher, level of involvement was based upon what Hagen had actually done, and included moderate personal contact over and above the written communications. The results were revealing.

The treatment that was based upon Hagen's actual performance resulted in the same average weight loss – 22 lb (5·5 kg). By contrast, the bibliotherapy conducted with truly minimal contact produced weight losses of no more than 6 lb (2·7 kg). These results suggest that the failure of three of the earlier studies to find differences between face-to-face treatment and bibliotherapy may have been the result of small but highly significant amounts of personal contact in the bibliotherapy regime. Such an outcome would not detract from the practical value of bibliotherapy in providing a more favourable cost/effectiveness ratio than traditional face-to-face encounters, and it provides a useful paradigm for a fine-grain analysis of the form and function of the doctor–patient relationship.

New directions in treatment
New directions in treatment have developed in the shadow of increasing awareness that a major problem plagues the behavioural treatment of obesity: despite a vast amount of clinical application and considerable research, the results of behavioural treatment for obesity have improved little in the 10 years since the method's introduction. It appears that the effectiveness of this treatment has reached its limits. What has been the response to this impasse? To date, the impasse has not been widely recognized, and suggestions for resolving it have been few. One of the most promising new measures has been to combine non-behavioural and behavioural techniques. So far two such combinations have been assessed: behaviour modification with diet and behaviour modification with medication.

The 'protein-sparing-modified-fast' utilized in the first study was that developed by Blackburn and his colleagues[43] and contained 1·4 g of high quality protein per kg of lean body mass. Its three meals a day contained 270–700 kcal in the form of protein hydrolysate or protein-lean meat, fish, or fowl, with supplements of vitamins and minerals.

The first phase of the programme consisted of an evaluation period, during which patients ate their usual foods, recorded their intake in a food diary, measured their physical activity with a pedometer and were introduced to behavioural principles in a classroom setting. The second, or diet, phase was introduced after patients had shown satisfactory progress in the first phase, usually after 2 or 3 weeks of treatment. After a prolonged period devoted primarily to the protein-sparing-modified-fast and to increasing physical activity, dietary restrictions were liberalized. Vegetables were introduced first, followed by fruit. Finally, the patient returned to a balanced diet which restricted only concentrated carbohydrates. During this third, termination, phase, group sessions were held to teach a more detailed behavioural programme. The responsibility for continuation of the programme was gradually shifted from staff-management to self-management.

Treatment was of an intensity and duration unprecedented in the literature on outpatient treatment of obesity by any modality. During the first 2 weeks, patients were seen daily. Then frequency was decreased to once a week for the duration of the programme. Average duration of treatment was 28 weeks and a vigorous effort was made to reduce all patients to their desirable weight during that time. The absence of control groups makes it difficult to determine the extent to which the results of treatment were a consequence of the character of this treatment or of its duration. This uncertainty is disappointing, for the results of the Lindner and Blackburn study are impressive. In one of their two clinics, mean weight fell from 206 to 151 lb (93·6 to 68·6 kg), and a majority of patients are said to have maintained this loss. The results in the other clinic, reported only in terms of the Trulson, Walsh and Caso criteria[44] also seem to have been excellent.

A second approach that may increase the effectiveness of behaviour modification is to combine it with pharmacotherapy. The most ambitious such effort was a large-scale randomized clinical trial of four treatments of 140 moderate to severely obese people[45]. These treatments were:

1. routine medical treatment with a common anti-obesity medication – fenfluramine – in a doctor's office;
2. behaviour modification carried out in groups of ten according to a standard protocol[20];
3. fenfluramine given in a group discussion format with monetary deposits to foster attendance; and

4. fenfluramine combined with behaviour modification in groups identical to regime 2.

Average weight losses over a period of 6 months for the four treatments were 14, 23, 10, and 32 lb (6·4, 10·5, 13·6, 14·5 kg) respectively. There was an average 4 lb (1·8 kg) weight gain in a no-treatment control group. A low dropout rate increases the confidence which these figures inspire.

This study has significance beyond what it shows about behavioural control of obesity; for it shows that the manner in which it is administered can greatly influence the effectiveness of medication – from a mean weight loss of 14 lb (6·4 kg) in the doctor's office to 30 lb (13·6 kg) in a group format. The efficacy of a group format had been reported previously, but not to this degree[35]. It brings into question the conventional wisdom that medication is of little benefit in the treatment of obesity.

A follow-up of this study is in progress and the first 6 months' findings have tempered the first enthusiasm. Patients receiving behaviour-modification alone (treatment 2) lost a further 3 lb (1·4 kg) to reach a weight 26 lb (11·8 kg) below that at the beginning of treatment. However, a weight *gain* of 10 lb (4·5 kg) occurred not only in the fenfluramine-alone conditions but also in the combined behaviour modification/fenfluramine condition. Apparently weight lost by medication is readily regained, even when patients have learned the traditional behaviour modification procedures. This finding has prompted a new look at the maintenance of weight lost by behavioural techniques, a topic that has been the subject of a recent review[46].

Maintenance of weight loss
Before behaviour modification was introduced, effective maintenance of weight loss was as uncommon as was effective weight loss. The greater losses behavioural measures achieved raised hopes that these losses might be better maintained[47]. After all, they had apparently resulted from changes in eating behaviour, which might be maintained, rather than from traditional drug and diet therapy, which had made no pretensions to effecting long-term changes. Early reports seemed to confirm these hopes; the study with the greatest weight losses also apparently showed effective mainten-ance of losses for at least a year[37]. A recent comprehensive review, how-ever, has questioned this early optimism[46]. In some studies, what had appeared as effective maintenance of weight loss was actually a statistical artifact. When weight losses were maintained those losses tended to have been trivial. Behaviour modification may produce somewhat better main-tenance of weight loss than is achieved by traditional measures, but the results leave much to be desired.

The unsatisfactory maintenance of weight loss must be considered in the light of the processes involved in behaviour therapy. Bandura has recently suggested that effective behaviour therapy involves three logically distinct and often operationally separable processes; *induction* of the change, its *generalization,* and its *maintenance*[48-49]. There is no reason for the contingencies affecting one process to be the same as those affecting the other two. Some of the problems traditionally approached by behaviour therapy have involved primarily the induction and generalization of change as, for example, in the systematic desensitization of patients with phobias. In phobic patients, the freedom from anxiety and the broadened scope of social activities that result from therapy may be sufficient reward to maintain the altered behaviour with no further effort. Changing eating behaviour is a very different problem. Induction and generalization of eating behaviours prescribed in programmes of the type described here are not particularly difficult to achieve and, as we have noted, these programmes have produced greater weight loss than have a variety of alternate treatments. But reducing weight has minimal effects upon anxiety, and the somewhat greater social activities that weight loss promotes are limited bulwarks against the inducements to eat that bombard the dieter and stimulate eating. And they are no match for the powerful biological rewards of satiety that follow eating. A simple analysis of these behavioural contingencies would make it easy to predict that changes in eating behaviour would be extraordinarily difficult to maintain.

On both empirical and theoretical grounds, it thus appears that a major problem in the behavioural control of obesity is the maintenance of changes in eating behaviour and in resultant weight loss. And a major challenge is the development of strategies specifically designed to achieve maintenance of behaviour change and of weight loss.

To date, several studies have been directed to this end. In one study, Brownell incorporated behavioural treatment measures into a training programme for couples[27]. Earlier reports had suggested that such an approach might be fruitful. Stuart and Davis[15] had found from an analysis of mealtime interactions that spouses might exert either a favourable or an unfavourable influence on the efforts of a group of wives to lose weight. The Mahoneys[26] noted a high correlation between indices of social support within the family and weight lost during treatment.

Brownell developed a behavioural programme in which a married couple, rather than an individual, was the focus of a variety of behavioural techniques, including mutual monitoring of food-related behaviours, stimulus control, modelling, and reinforcement[27]. For each part of the patients' programme there was a corresponding part for the spouses, who participated fully in each training session. Here they were taught to model appropriate eating behaviours such as slowing eating by putting down the fork between bites, 'to set a good example'. Similarly they learned specific ways of engaging the patient during times of temptation in activities incompatible with eating. Each partner monitored the other partner's behaviour as well as his/her own. The programme stressed that mutual effort was critical to success.

Although this has been assessed to date by only one study, this study was well enough designed, and its results sufficiently decisive, that the approach must be regarded as promising. It was compared with two other treatments in which patients received substantially the same programme, except as individuals rather than as couples. In one treatment regime patients had spouses deemed 'cooperative', or at least as cooperative as those who took part in the couples training programme, as evidenced by their reported willingness to take part in such a programme. In the other treatment spouses had been deemed 'uncooperative', as evidenced by their unwillingness to take part in such a programme – patients whose spouses had refused, in fact, to participate. Treatment occurred once weekly for $1\frac{1}{2}$ h, over a period of 10 weeks, followed by once-monthly treatments for the next 6 months. A \$50 deposit, return of which was contingent upon attendance, not weight loss, helped eliminate dropouts altogether. Patients consisted of 10 men and 19 women, averaging 56% overweight.

All groups lost weight. At the end of the 10-week treatment programme losses were 20 lb (9·1 kg) for the couples training programme, 15 lb (6·8 kg) for the 'cooperative-spouse-patient-alone' treatment and 12 lb (5·5 kg) for the 'uncooperative-spouse-patient-alone' treatment (see Figure 7). These differences did not quite reach statistical significance, but 6 months later weight loss of the couples training group reached 30 lb (13·6 kg), which was significantly greater than the losses of the individual patient groups – 19 and 15 lb (8·6 and 6·8 kg) each. The couples training approach to maintenance of weight lost in behavioural treatment seems sufficiently promising that a large-scale effort to replicate this study is already under way and the results should soon be available[50].

A second innovative approach to maintenance of weight loss has been proposed by Bandura and Simon[51] who have used monitoring of the number of mouthfuls of food consumed as the basis for setting very short-term goals. Small weight gains during the period after the end of formal treatment are used as an early warning system to trigger the reintroduction of this 'proximal-goal procedure'.

Booster sessions have also been proposed as a method of improving maintenance. In many behavioural programmes, booster sessions are routinely scheduled after weekly treatment sessions end, yet the evidence indicates that booster sessions are no more effective than no boosters. Kingsley and Wilson[35] and Ashby and Wilson[52] found that booster sessions were not effective for subjects receiving group behavioural treatment, although in the first study booster sessions were effective for subjects

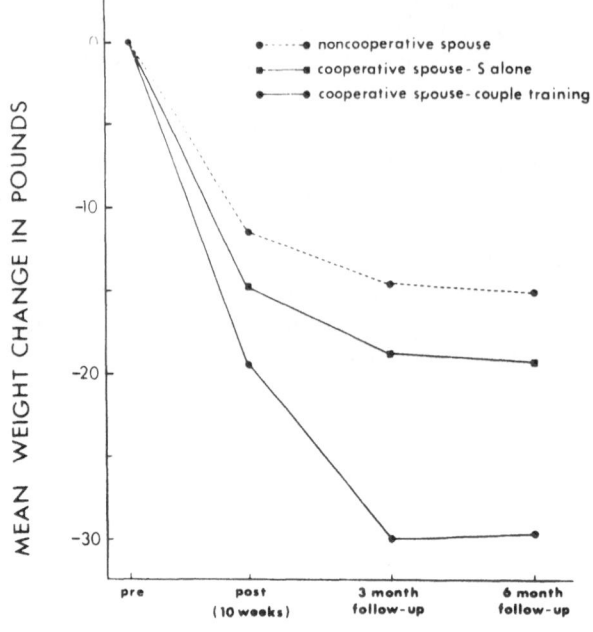

TIME OF ASSESSMENT

Figure 7   Mean weight changes during treatment and follow-up for the three spouse conditions. From Brownell *et al.*[27]

in individual treatment[35]. Several recent studies have also failed to support the notion that booster sessions assist in the maintenance of weight loss[26,45,53].

NON-PROFESSIONAL WEIGHT REDUCTION GROUPS

Health care needs have increased so rapidly in recent years that they threaten to outdistance the supply of physicians and medical facilities. A major response to the mounting pressures for health care has been the reorganization of traditional systems of delivery of medical care and increased use of paramedical personnel. In the face of our pressing health needs, one source of assistance has received curiously little attention from the medical profession: the self-help group. The most widely known of these groups is Alcoholics Anonymous (AA), but individuals have organized to help themselves with problems as varied as psychosis, ileostomy and narcotics addiction. The largest number of persons engaged in self-help or non-professional activities, however, are those who have joined together for the control of obesity. In the United States alone, over one million obese people a week take part in group efforts at weight reduction under lay auspices. Yet recent surveys show that only a very small minority of such persons – estimated at from 0 to 7% – have been referred by their physicians. This limited enthusiasm of the medical professional is not shared by many non-medical groups involved in health care, and a growing number of such persons are turning with increasing enthusiasm to non-medical organizations for the control of obesity. Thus, Stuart reports that 90% of persons attending a conference on behavioural medicine said that they believed that self-help groups were the treatment of choice for mild to moderate obesity and only 10% favoured medical auspices[54]. It is true that only 11% of this group were physicians, and psychologists constituted over half of its membership. Nevertheless, it is apparent that more and more persons are turning to self-help groups for weight control, and it behoves the physician to know something about these organizations. What can we say about them?

The rationale for the use of self-help groups is indisputable. Rapidly rising health costs have produced little improvement in health indices[55] and the public and the profession alike are aware of the paradox expressed by the title of the recent book by Knowles: *Doing Better and Feeling Worse: Health in the United States*[56]. If it were possible to shift a major burden of health care from the physician to the patient (and the control of body weight seems an excellent starting point) it might be possible to achieve better effects at lower costs. If professional guidance can improve the results of such lay efforts, it could be a most effective use of professional time. Some enthusiasts for the self-help movement see precisely such potential. Gartner and Reissman[57] see self-help groups as 'sometimes a complement or a supplement, sometimes an alternative, and sometimes a way of expanding and enriching professional practice, but rarely do they replace the professional where the professional's expertise is appropriate'.

Stuart[58] notes the 'formidable' benefits of self-help groups as:

1. they tend to maintain a specific task orientation;
2. they infuse a kind of faith in their programmes that builds motivation;
3. they are sufficiently informal to permit members to meet social needs – a factor that may strongly reinforce perseverence;
4. their peer leaders serve as role models for members;
5. they offer ready entry and withdrawal so that members can easily avail themselves of service when needed;
6. they help to 'normalize' their target behaviours so that members can mobilize their problem-solving capacities;
7. their self-help character allows members to attribute changes to personal growth, increasing the likelihood that these changes will be maintained;

8. they rely upon the effective principles of social marketing[59] so they can publicize and package their programmes in an appealing manner; and
9. their comparatively modest fees permit members to pay for the services they receive without reliance upon third-party payment which may undermine individual responsibility.

Stuart concludes that 'self-help programmes offer the advantage of an attractive, available, cost effective service for selected problems'[58].

The theoretical rationale for the use of self-help groups in the control of obesity is clear. So also is the remarkable acceptance of such programmes, as measured by the numbers of persons making use of their services. Although there is frequently a discrepancy between the number of persons said to join such a group and those actually attending sessions on a regular basis, it appears that well over two million persons a year join weight control programmes in the United States and that as many as one million persons may be making use of their services at any one time. Furthermore, these numbers appear to be growing.

Thus, from the point of view both of theoretical rationale and public acceptance, self-help groups have well established reasons for existence. But what are their practical results? What can the physician expect if he recommends such a programme for his patient? Here the results are less clear.

The TOPS Studies

The most intensively studied of the self-help groups is TOPS (Take Off Pounds Sensibly), and the potential and the problems of such organizations have perhaps been best elucidated in this group[1,60]. TOPS is a non-profit organization founded in 1948 by Esther Manz, a Milwaukee housewife who continues as its leader. There are reported to be 350 000 members organized in over 12 000 chapters, largely confined to the United States. The dominant characteristic of the members – and one with which TOPS shares with other lay groups – is its almost exclusively female membership; less than 1% are men. Average age of the members is 42, and their average weight is 188 lb (85·5 kg), which, with an average ideal weight of 119 lb (54·1 kg) makes them 58% overweight. Socio-economic status is largely lower-middle class. The annual fee is £5·2 for the first 2 years, falling to £4·0; this is the total cost of the programme to a member.

The meeting of a TOPS chapter lasts from 1½ to 2 h and is held once a week. It is under the direction of a woman who is elected leader for a 1-year period. The first of the essential activities is the weigh-in, which occurs before the formal start of the meeting. Each member is weighed in turn by an official, the weight recorder, on a set of professional scales. Many members feel that this monitoring is the most effective part of the TOPS programme.

The second of the essential activities is the announcement of each member's weight change during the past week. Only the number of pounds gained or lost is reported, never the person's actual weight, a practice designed to prevent discouragement of the heavier members of the group. As the weight change of each member is announced to the expectant group, responses characteristic of that group are made. A woman who has lost weight is invariably applauded and often receives other forms of approval. The one who has lost the most weight during the past week is designated as 'Queen' and may have a crown placed upon her head. The announcement of weight gain elicits a more varied response, extending from jeering, to silence, to expressions of sympathy. Although the practice is said to have declined in recent years, a hallmark of early TOPS meetings was the designation of the member who had gained the most weight as 'Pig of the Week' and her banishment to a symbolic pig pen.

The rest of the meeting is devoted to discussion, largely about dieting, competition between individuals for weight loss and singing from the extensive list of TOPS inspirational songs.

Successive steps in weight reduction are rewarded by bracelet charms and other artifacts, and members who reach their recommended weight are rewarded with a special ceremony and membership in KOPS (Keep Off Pounds Sensibly).

TOPS has perhaps the most favourable attitude towards the medical profession of any of the self-help groups, requiring that its members consult their personal physicians for estimation of goal weights and for prescription of reducing diets.

What are the results of the TOPS programme? At first glance, they appear impressive. A survey of 21 chapters carried out by the use of chapter records in 1968 showed a mean weight loss of 15 lb (6·8 kg) with a standard deviation of 15 lb (6·8 kg) and 2 years later a re-survey of these chapters showed a mean weight loss of 14 lb (6·4 kg) with a standard deviation of 17 lb (7·7 kg)[62]. Furthermore the percentages of persons losing more than 20 lb (9·1 kg), were 29 and 29, respectively, while the percentage of those losing more than 40 lb (18·2 kg) were 6·4 and 7·8, respectively.

Impressive as these figures seem, they must be regarded with caution; for they were the result of surveys of all persons in the organization at any one time. TOPS, as well as other self-help organizations, have very high dropout rates, and furthermore, those dropping out of treatment are likely to be persons with smallest weight losses. Thus, any cross-sectional assessment of treatment results will show weight losses which are increased by virtue of the dropout of less successful members. The extent of this effect depends directly upon the extent of the dropout rate. As a result, valid estimates of the weight losses achieved by self-help groups can be obtained only by cohort studies which consider all persons entering a programme and their weight loss at the time that they leave it. Unfortunately, no such study has yet been carried out.

A careful assessment of the dropout rate of persons in the TOPS chapters under study has shown that attrition rates of 47% at 1 year and 70% at 2[60]. High as these rates seem, they are the lowest yet reported for any self-help group, and are significantly lower than the 67% attrition rate at 1 year reported for TOPS when the records were kept by professional personnel in a later study[1].

Commercial weight-reduction groups

There have been a number of reports of commercial weight reduction groups, but they have tended to be long on explication and short on data. The most striking aspect of the results that have been reported has been the very high rates of dropout from treatment. These dropout rates are so high as to render suspect the weight losses that have been reported from the various programmes. They represent the results of that minority of persons who survived in the programme. Figure 8, adapted from Ashwell[61] shows that the TOPS attrition rate described above is the lowest of any reported, and far lower than those reported by commercial weight reduction groups. Attention should be paid to the curve labelled X/USA which describes the results of the most intensive study yet undertaken of dropout rates from weight reduction programmes. Nash[62] found that by the time she carried out this study, in the mid-1970s, members joining this commercial weight reduction programme had joined an average of three times previously, and that the number of previous memberships was highly correlated with dropping out of treatment. By contrast, the few other characteristics predictive of attrition were of considerably less importance: for example, persons who believed that they lacked information about food and nutrition tended to stay in treatment longer. (This factor may have interacted with previous membership in the group, since such knowledge was acquired in the course of previous meetings. Once this information had become acquired the incentive to stay in the group was lost.)

The largest of the commercial weight reduction organizations, and, in fact, the largest of any such organization, is Weight Watchers, which was founded in 1963 by another overweight housewife, Jean Neditch. Upon joining members pay a small registration fee and then a weekly class fee of about £1·5. Members who reach their goal weight are eligible to attend monthly classes without charge for life, so long as they remain within 2 lb of their goal weight and do not miss a monthly meeting.

The Weight Watchers format owes much to TOPS, including the weekly

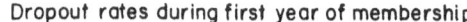

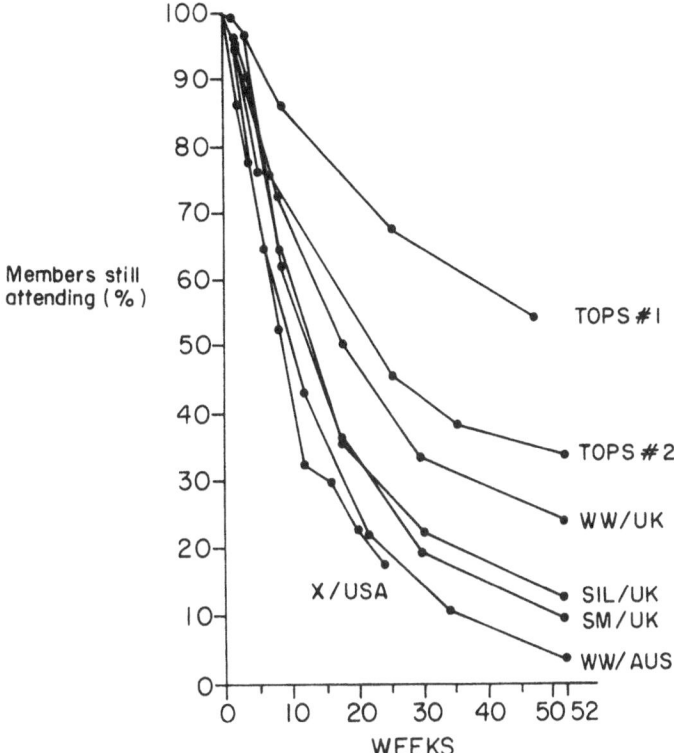

Figure 8 Proportion of members still attending at intervals of up to 1 year after first joining. Groups are from the United Kingdom, the United States, and Australia. The groups are Take Off Pounds Sensibly (TOPS), Weight Watchers (WW), Silhouette Slimming Clubs (SIL), Slimming Magazine Slimming Clubs (SM) and an unidentified group (X). TOPS data are from an initial study of the organization[60] (TOPS No. 1), and from a later study by the same group[1] (TOPS No. 2). From Ashwell[61]

weigh-in and the group support. Weight Watchers, however, introduced two significant new measures. First was a palatable, satisfying and well-structured diet (based upon sound nutritional principles) that provides enough food to preclude hunger. The second measure was the introduction of a paid lecturer who provided the basic information about the programme. These lecturers were selected from among persons who had successfully completed the Weight Watchers programme, and they are usually highly effective speakers and often have charismatic personalities. These two measures have increased the structure of the group meetings as well as helping to structure the eating behaviour of the participants; both are characteristics which should improve the effectiveness of the programme.

What can we say about the effectiveness of commercial weight-loss groups in terms of the essential measure of weight loss? The most comprehensive survey has been prepared by Ashwell[61] who made extensive use of the earlier survey which she had carried out with Garrow[63]. Table 1, adapted from Ashwell, shows some characteristics of the three United Kingdom (UK) groups which she surveyed together with two of the American groups described above and one Australian group reported by Williams and Duncan[66-67]. Ashwell's figures of weight loss must be

Table 1 Characteristics of commercial and self-help weight reduction groups in the United Kingdom, the United States, and Australia. The groups are Weight Watchers (WW), Slimming Magazine Slimming Clubs (SM), Silhouette Slimming Club (SIL), Take Off Pounds Sensibly (TOPS), and an unidentified group (X). From Ashwell[61]

| | United Kingdom | | | United States | | Australia |
	WW	SM	SIL	TOPS	X	WW
Number of chapters	800	420	1000	12000	—*	—
Mean age of members	36	39	35	42	—	—
Starting weight (kg)	80	79	74	85	80	78
Cost per visit (£)	1·3	0·8	0·7	0	1·7	1·9
Reported attainment of ideal weight (%)	28	20	31	—	—	22
Cost per kg (£)†	2·6	1·6	1·2	0·6	—	4·4
Percentage referred by MD	2	3	0	3	—	7

* Not reported

† Calculated from [membership fee + (n weekly fee)] ÷ weight loss (kg), where n = average length of membership in weeks

qualified not only by the very high attrition rates shown in Figure 8 but also by the fact that her data on weight loss are responses to a questionnaire based upon no more than a 57% response rate. There is strong reason to believe that responders are biased towards more effective weight losers.

The lowest weight loss reported in Ashwell's survey is from TOPS, with a mean 14·5 lb (6·6 kg), and the highest loss is the 30 lb (11·8 kg) which was reported for UK Weight Watchers. It is possible that the most reliable data in an unreliable set are those of Williams and Duncan, who compared the results of Weight Watchers classes in Australia with those in a hospital obesity clinic[64-65]. The women in the Weight Watchers group are reported to have lost 18 lb (8·2 kg), while those in the hospital programme lost 9·2 lb (4·2 kg). It should be noted that the subjects were not randomly assigned to the two programmes, and this comparison was in no sense a randomized clinical trial.

A therapeutic coalition: behaviour modification and patient self-help

The early results with behaviour modification suggested that it might be introduced with profit into self-help organizations. It seemed that behaviour modification might provide self-help organizations with a more effective treatment technology, while self-help organizations could provide a means for the widespread application of behaviour modification. A large-scale controlled clinical trial to assess this possibility was carried out by Levitz and Stunkard[1].

Four treatment conditions were applied to each of four TOPS chapters containing a total of 234 subjects. Treatments were:

1. behaviour modification conducted by a professional therapist;
2. behaviour modification conducted by the TOPS chapter leader;
3. nutrition education conducted by the TOPS leader; and
4. continuation of the usual TOPS programme.

Behaviour modification markedly increased the effectiveness of the TOPS programme, lowering attrition rates sharply and increasing weight loss. During the 3 months of active treatment fewer TOPS members dropped out of the two behaviour modification groups than out of the nutrition education and the control groups. At 9 months follow-up this difference had become striking. Only 38% and 41% had dropped out of the behaviour modification groups, compared with 55% and 67% for the nutrition education and the control groups respectively ($\chi^2 = 12\cdot35$, $P < 0\cdot01$).

Such differential attrition rates seriously biased the results against behaviour modification; decreasing attrition means retaining less successful members. Despite this bias, behaviour modification groups lost significantly more weight than those in the control regimes ($F = 11\cdot7$, $P < \cdot001$). The chapters in which behaviour modification was introduced by a professional therapist lost 4·2 lb (1·9 kg), significantly more than the weight loss in either the nutrition education ($-0\cdot22$ lb, $-0\cdot1$ kg) or the TOPS control group, in which subjects actually gained 0·66 lb (0·3 kg). The chapters in which behaviour modification was introduced by professional therapists lost significantly more weight than those taught the same programme by the TOPS chapter leaders (-2 lb, $-0\cdot9$ kg).

At a 9-month follow-up these differences had become even greater. Subjects in the behaviour modification groups led by professionals not only maintained their higher weight loss but even increased it to 5·7 lb (2·6 kg). The initial weight loss of subjects in the behaviour modification programme conducted by TOPS chapter leaders was not maintained during follow-up, and the subjects' weights returned to pre-treatment levels. However, these subjects did better than the nutrition education and control groups which actually gained weight during follow-up (+2·9 lb, 1·3 kg, and 4 lb, 1·8 kg, respectively).

These results, modest as they were, were still decisive enough to show that behaviour modification could significantly improve the effectiveness of TOPS. The carefully monitored data from this study may prove to be a closer approximation to the results of these groups than the more optimistic figures which are presented by the organizations themselves. Be that as it may, the logic of combining behaviour modification and patient self-help was sufficiently compelling that it was not long before Weight Watchers began to incorporate behaviour modification as a key element of its programme.

The programme (designed by Stuart) consists of a series of 'modules', or printed instruction sheets, each of which contains the rationale for several specific steps aimed at self-management, as well as charts for members recording their progress in taking these steps. The 18 modules contain recommendations for coping with mood-triggered eating, for slowing the rate of eating, for differentiating between hunger and appetite, for arranging environments that facilitate constructive eating, for reprogramming social interactions related to eating, and a variety of other behavioural instructions. After preparation and pre-testing of the modules, training materials were prepared to help the lecturers use them effectively. These materials included a detailed explanation of the logic of each module through modelling, audio and video tapes of successful model presentations and cue cards for lecturers used in conducting classes. Lecturers make every attempt to stimulate the maximum possible interaction among members and to build their commitment to the recommended techniques. As might be imagined, the introduction of a programme of this scope and complexity to the lecturers of 13 000 programmes (in the United States alone) has been no small task, and the results are doubtless somewhat mixed. Nevertheless, the introduction of these programmes means that behavioural treatment for obesity is now being provided to half a million persons a week in the United States alone. Surely this constitutes a major social movement, and one whose consequences have still to be appreciated.

Although rigorous evaluation of the results of the behavioural component of the Weight Watchers programme has not been reported, a quasi-experiment involving samples of 2000 or more members has been reported. During a 12-week test, persons receiving the traditional programme lost an average of 1·1 lb (0·5 kg) per week, while those in the behavioural programme lost 1·3 lb (0·5 kg). When only very frequent attenders were considered, these values increased to 1·3 lb (0·6 kg) and 1·5 lb (0·7 kg) per week[58]. Attrition rates in the different treatments were not reported.

Overview of non-professional groups
How are we to view this large and unruly new element which has entered

the field of treatment of obesity ? First, as we have noted, the theoretical rationale for a self-help approach to weight control is unexceptional and the large and growing popular demand makes it clear that the approach is a popular one. We are still very much in the dark about the results of such efforts, however, and a growing disinclination on the part of these organizations to subject themselves to objective scrutiny makes it unlikely that such evidence will soon be available. Nevertheless, orthodox medical treatment is not sufficiently effective to justify ignoring any potential assistance. It may well be that most efforts at weight reduction are primarily personal matters, and that outside influences such as the physician or the self-help group provide no more than the stimulus which triggers the ensuing effort. The economy of the self-help groups makes them particularly attractive as such a stimulus.

There is reason to believe that the results of self-help groups, if not as good as their proponents maintain, are still as good as the results of the usual treatment carried out in the doctor's office. If this be the case, then an important new resource for the physician is at hand. For these treatments are economical, readily accessible, highly supportive and capable of conveying important nutritional and behavioural information.

References

1 Levitz, L. S. and Stunkard, A. J. (1974). A therapeutic coalition for obesity: Behavior modification and patient self-help. *Am. J. Psychiatry*, **131**, 423

2 Stunkard, A. J. (1958). The management of obesity. *NY J. Med.*, **58**, 79

3 Stunkard, A. J. and McLaren-Hume, M. (1959). The results of treatment for obesity. *Arch. Intern. Med.*, **103**, 79

4 Shipman, W. G. and Plessat, M. R. (1963). Anxiety and depression in obese dieters. *Arch. Gen. Psychiatry*, **8**, 530

5 Feinstein, A. R. (1959). The measurement of success in weight reduction: An analysis of methods and new index. *J. Chronic Dis.*, **10**, 439

6 Feinstein, A. R. (1960). The treatment of obesity: an analysis of methods, results, and factors which influence success. *J. Chronic Dis.*, **11**, 349

7 Stunkard, A. J. and Rush, A. J. (1974). Dieting and depression reexamined: A critical view of reports of untoward response during weight reduction for obesity. *Ann. Intern. Med.*, **81**, 526

8 Stuart, R. B. (1967). Behavioral control of overeating. *Behav. Res. Ther.*, **5**, 357

9 Stunkard, A. J. (1975). From explanation to action in psychosomatic medicine: the case of obesity. *Psychosom. Med.*, **37**, 195

10 Wilson, G. T. (1978). Methodological considerations in treatment outcome research on obesity. *J. Consult. Clin. Psychol.*, **46**, 687

11 Abramson, E. E. (1977). Behavioral approaches to weight control: an updated review. *Behav. Res. Ther.*, **15**, 355

12 Stunkard, A. J. and Mahoney, M. J. (1976). Behavioral treatment of eating disorders. In H. Leitenberg (ed.). *The Handbook of Behavior Modification.* (Englewood Cliffs, N.J.: Prentice-Hall)

13 Leon, G. R. (1976). Current directions in the treatment of obesity. *Psychol. Bull.*, **83**, 557

14 Jeffery, R. W., Wing, R. R. and Stunkard, A. J. (1978). Behavioral treatment of obesity: The state of the art in 1978. *Behav. Ther.*, **9,** 189

15 Stuart, R. B. and Davis, B. (1972). *Slim Chance in a Fat World: Behavioural Control of Obesity.* (Champaign: Research Press)

16 Foreyt, J. P. (ed.). (1977). *Behavioral Treatments of Obesity.* (New York: Pergamon)

17 Stuart, R. B. (1971). A three-dimensional approach for the treatment of obesity. *Behav. Res. Ther.*, **9,** 177

18 Ferster, C. B., Nurnberger, J. I. and Levitt, E. B. (1962). The control of eating. *J. Mathetics*, **1,** 87

19 Mahoney, M. J. and Mahoney, K. (1976). *Permanent Weight Control: A Total Solution to the Dieter's Dilemma.* (New York: Norton)

20 Ferguson, J. F. (1975). *Learning to Eat: Behavior Modification for Weight Control.* (Palo Alto, Calif.: Bull)

21 Kazdin, A. E. (1974). Self-monitoring and behavior change. In M. J. Mahoney and C. C. Thoresen (eds.). *Self-control: Power to the Person.* (Monterey, Calif.: Brooks-Cole)

22 Mahoney, M. J., Moura, N. G. M. and Wade, T. C. (1973). The relative efficacy of self-reward, self-punishment, and self-monitoring techniques for weight loss. *J. Consult. Clin. Psychol.*, **40,** 404

23 Stollak, G. E. (1967). Weight loss obtained under different experimental procedures. *Psychotherapy: Theory, Research and Practice*, **4,** 61

24 Romanczyk, R. G. (1974). Self-monitoring in the treatment of obesity: Parameters of reactivity. *Behav. Ther.*, **5,** 531

25 Wilson, G. T. and Brownell, K. D. (1978). Behavior therapy for obesity: Including family members in the treatment process. *Behav. Ther.* (In press)

26 Mahoney, M. J. and Mahoney, K. (1976). Treatment of obesity: A clinical exploration. In B. J. Williams, S. Martin and J. P. Foreyt (eds.). *Obesity: Behavioral Approaches to Dietary Management.* (New York: Brunner/Mazel)

27 Brownell, K. D., Heckerman, C. L., Westlake, R. J. Hayes, S. C. and Monti, P. M. (1978). The effect of couples training and partner cooperativeness in the behavioral treatment of obesity. *Behav. Res. Ther.* (In press)

28 Jeffrey, D. B. (1974). A comparison of the effects of external control and self-control on the modification and maintenance of weight. *J. Abnorm. Psychol.*, **83,** 404

29 Mahoney, M. J. (1974). *Cognition and Behavior Modification.* (Cambridge, Mass.: Ballinger)

30 Meichenbaum, D. (1977). *Cognitive Behavior Modification: An Integrative Approach.* (New York: Plenum)

31 Naughton, J. P. and Hellerstein, H. K. (eds.). (1973). *Exercise Testing and Exercise Training in Coronary Heart Disease.* (New York: Academic Press)

32 Brownell, K. D., Albaum, J. M. and Stunkard, A. J. (1978). Evaluation and modification of activity patterns in the natural environment. (Manuscript submitted for publication)

33 Paul, G. L. (1966). *Insight Vs. Desensitization in Psychotherapy: An Experiment in Anxiety Reduction.* (Stanford, Calif.: Stanford University Press)

34 Harris, M. G. (1969). Self-directed program for weight control: A pilot study. *J. Abnorm. Psychol.*, **74,** 263

35 Kingsley, R. B. and Wilson, G. T. (1977). Behavior therapy for obesity: A comparative investigation of long-term efficacy. *J. Consult. Clin. Psychol.*, **45,** 288

36 Wollersheim, J. P. (1970). Effectiveness of group therapy based on learning

principles in the treatment of overweight women. *J. Abnorm. Psychol.*, **76**, 462

37 Penick, S. B., Filion, R., Fox, S. and Stunkard, A. J. (1971). Behavior modification in the treatment of obesity. *Psychosom. Med.*, **33**, 49

38 Hagen, R. L. (1974). Group therapy versus bibliotherapy in weight reduction. *Behav. Ther.*, **5**, 222

39 Ferstl, R., Jokusch, V. and Brengelman, J. C. (1975). Die verhaltenstherapeutische Behandlung des Ubergewichts. *Int. J. Health Educ.*, **18**, 119

40 Hanson, R. W., Borden, B. L., Hall, S. M. and Hall, R. G. (1976). Use of programmed instruction in teaching self-management skills to overweight adults. *Behav. Ther.*, **7**, 366

41 Brownell, K. D., Heckerman, C. L. and Westlake, R. J. (1978). Therapist and group contact as variables in the behavioral treatment of obesity. *J. Consult. Clin. Psychol.*, **46**, 593

42 Fernan, W. S. (1973). The role of experimenter contact in behavioral bibliotherapy of obesity. Unpublished manuscript, Pennsylvania State University

43 Lindner, P. G. and Blackburn, G. L. (1976). An interdisciplinary approach to obesity utilizing fasting modified by protein-sparing therapy. *Obesity/Bariatric Med.*, **5**, 198

44 Trulson, M., Walsh, E. D. and Caso, E. K. (1947). A study of obese patients in a nutrition clinic. *J. Am. Diet. Assoc.*, **23**, 941

45 Stunkard, A. J., Craighead, L. W. and O'Brien, R. (1978). New treatments for obesity. Paper presented at the *Annual Meeting of the American Psychiatric Association*, May, Atlanta

46 Stunkard, A. J. and Penick, S. B. (1978). Behavior modification in the treatment of obesity: The problem of maintaining weight loss. *Arch. Gen. Psychiatry*. (In press)

47 Stunkard, A. J. (1972). New therapies for the eating disorders. *Arch. Gen. Psychiatry*, **26**, 391

48 Bandura, A. (1969). *Principles of Behavior Modification*. (New York: Holt, Rinehart & Winston)

49 Bandura, A. (1977). *Social Learning Theory*. (Englewood Cliffs, N.J.: Prentice-Hall)

50 Brownell, K. D., Cook, L. G. and Stunkard, A. J. (1978). Spouse intervention and pharmacological therapy as methods of enhancing magnitude and maintenance of weight loss. (In preparation)

51 Bandura, A. and Simon, K. M. (1977). The role of proximal intentions in self-regulation of refractory behavior. *Cognitive Ther. Res.*, **1**, 177

52 Ashby, W. A. and Wilson, G. T. (1977). Behavior therapy for obesity: booster sessions and long-term maintenance of weight loss. *Behav. Res. Ther.*, **15**, 451

53 Polly, S. J. and Kelnan, C. A., (1976). Self-Management training with various booster treatments: effects on the modification and maintenance of weight. Paper presented at the *Annual Meeting of the Association for the Advancement of Behaviour Therapy*, December, New York

54 Stuart, R. B. and Mitchell, C. A. (1978). A professional and a consumer perspective on self-help weight control groups. *Psychiatric Clinics of North America*. (In press)

55 Kristein, M. M., Arnold, C. B. and Wynder, E. L. (1977). Health economics and preventive care. *Science*, **195**, 457

56 Knowles, J. D. (1977). *Doing Better and Feeling Worse*. (New York: Norton).

57 Gartner, A. and Reissman, F. (1977). *Self-help in the Human Services*. (San Francisco: Jossey-Bass).

58 Stuart, R. B. (1977). Self-help for self-management. In R. B. Stuart (ed.). *Behavioral Self-management.* (New York: Brunner/Mazel)

59 Kolter, P. and Zaltman, G. (1971). Social marketing: An approach to planned social change. *J. Marketing,* **35,** 3

60 Garb, A. R. and Stunkard, A. J. (1974). Effectiveness of a self-help group in obesity control. *Arch. Intern. Med.,* **134,** 716

61 Ashwell, M. (1978). Commercial weight loss groups. In G. Bray (ed.), *Recent Advances in Obesity Research: II.* (London: Newman Publishing Co.). (In press)

62 Nash, J. D. (1977). Curbing drop-out from treatment for obesity. Unpublished dissertation, Stanford University

63 Ashwell, M. and Garrow, J. S. (1975). A survey of three slimming and weight control organizations in the UK. *Nutr.,* **29,** 347

64 Williams, A. E. and Duncan, B. A. (1976). A commercial weight reducing organization: A critical analysis. *Med. J. Aust.,* **1,** 781

65 Williams, A. E. and Duncan, B. A. (1976). Comparative results of an obesity clinic and weight reducing organization *Med. J. Aust.,* **1,** 800

Index

adipocyte *see* fat cell
adipose tissue
  as energy store, 3, 4
  loss due to exercise, 124, 126
adolescence, treatment of obesity in, 11, 12, 29
alcohol, in diabetes, 37
amphetamine
  anorexic action of, 56–7, 68–71
  clinical use of, 86–7
angina pectoris and obesity, 41
anorexia nervosa, 15, 104
anorexic drugs
  characteristics of, 56–8
  mechanism of action, 68–74
  testing of, 66; in man, 74–7
anti-obesity drugs, use of, 85–117
  see also anorexic drugs
appetite suppressants *see* anorexic drugs
apronectomy, as treatment of obesity, 166, 169

behaviour therapy, in treatment of obesity, 199–218
'bibliotherapy', 211–13
biguanides, anti-obesity drugs, 98–101
biliary tract disease, associated with obesity, 7
blood pressure, effect of exercise on, 127–8
  see also hypertension
bromocriptine, as anti-obesity agent, 103–4

bypass operations, as treatment of obesity
  gastric, 187–91
  small bowel (jejuno-ileal), 166–87

calculi, after bypass operations, 183–4
calorie intake
  effect of calorie density on, 23
  effect of fibre on, 23–4
  effect of meal frequency on, 22–3
  in diabetes, 36–7
carbohydrate
  desirable intake of, 24; in CHD, 42; in diabetes, 36
  low-carbohydrate diet, 24–5; in pregnancy, 33–4
cardiac failure *see* heart attack
cardiovascular disease, associated with obesity, 7, 41–3, 133
catecholamines, action of drugs on, 86–94
  see also dopamine, noradrenaline
CHD *see* coronary heart disease
children *see* infancy
chlorphentermine
  anorexic action, 56–7
  efficacy, 104–11
cholestyramine, as anti-obesity agent, 103
cigarette smoking, 19
CNS, role in feeding, 59–60
colon, in bypass operations, 168–71, 188
'compulsive eaters', 4, 5